WHAT TO DO IN A
GENERAL PRACTICE EMERGENCY

What to do in a general practice emergency

Melanie Darwent MA, BM, BCh, FRCS (Eng)
Specialist Registrar in Accident and Emergency, Oxford Region

Rosaleen Gregg BSC, MB BS, DCH, DRCOG, MRCGP
GP and Clinical Lecturer in General Practice at the Department
of General Practice and Primary Care, St Bartholomew's and the
Royal London School of Medicine and Dentistry, Queen Mary
and Westfield College, London

Ian Higginson BM, Dip Obst, Dip Paed, DFFP, MRCGP
GP and Accident and Emergency Registrar, currently working in
Australasia

Ed Peile MB BS, MRCS, MRCP, FRCGP, DRCOG, DCH
GP and GP Trainer, Aston Clinton, Buckinghamshire

The artwork is by Caroline Wilkinson, medical artist.

Collated by Ian Higginson. The *What to do in an Emergency* series
is edited by Ian Higginson and David Montgomery.

BMJ
Publishing
Group

First published in 1997
by the BMJ Publishing Group, BMA House, Tavistock Square,
London WC1H 9JR

British Library Cataloguing in Publication Data

A catalogue record for this book is available from the British Library

ISBN 0-7279-1183-X

Typeset, printed and bound in Great Britain
by Latimer Trend & Co. Ltd, Plymouth

Quick reference guide

Contents

Contents

Contents

Useful telephone numbers

Fill in your own details so that you have them handy.

Help: 999

Your surgery:

Ambulance control:

Local hospitals:

Duty Social Worker:

Out of hours District Nurses:

Emergency Midwifery number:

Local Poisons Unit:

Local Police:

Coroners Officer:

Others:

Acknowledgements

We are grateful for the help and advice we have received while developing this booklet. The drafts were read by many GPs and emergency care specialists, and their comments and criticism were invaluable in our attempts to produce a booklet that we hope is useful and relevant to its readers.

Valuable contributions were received from Hannah Buckley, Mike Corbett, Tony Higginson, Iain McNeil of BASICS, David Montgomery, Phil Munro, and Brendon Murphy.

We also received special help from Dr M Colquhoun and Dr A Handley of the Resuscitation Council, Dr B Harrison and Professor M Silverman of the British Thoracic Society, and Dr K Mackway-Jones of the Advanced Life Support Group.

We would like to thank the Resuscitation Council (UK) and the European Resuscitation Council for giving us permission to reproduce their resuscitation guidelines and the artwork on page 3.

A proportion of the royalties from this booklet is being donated to BASICS.

What to do in a General Practice Emergency is dedicated to the families of GPs, whose lives are so often disrupted when such emergencies arise.

Foreword

The concept of emergency care has developed rapidly in the last 10 years. All general practitioners should examine this aspect of their work to ensure the delivery of a high quality emergency service to their patients. Life threatening emergencies do not occur every day in general practice: some conditions such as anaphylactic shock may occur only a few times in a professional lifetime. The task of keeping up to date is a particular challenge because of the rarity of such events. This book should help GPs respond to this challenge and provides a quick reference source, when required, in the doctor's bag. For these reasons this book is both timely and necessary.

It is always encouraging when professionals of different disciplines work together. It is especially so when their cooperation results in a publication such as this. The authors have a background in general practice and accident and emergency care. They have described an approach to *What to do in a General Practice Emergency* using stepped treatment protocols which reflect practical aspects of resuscitation in the community. The intention has been to provide sensible guidance in a clear and easy to follow way, making use of diagrams and flow charts where appropriate. Emphasis is given to basic life support and practical procedures.

Recognition of the need to triage at the site of multiple casualties, the importance of good record keeping, and the need to look after yourself, both mentally and physically, are also well covered. General practitioners also need to be properly equipped for emergency care. They must carry a suitable range of drugs for the emergencies they are likely to face. The traditional black bag should now be accompanied by a range of items, which may include a nebuliser, intravenous fluids, an electrocardiograph machine, and a defibrillator. "What to carry in your doctor's bag" is clearly an important section.

The authors are particularly well placed to guide the reader. Perhaps, more importantly, they are experienced in day to day clinical care so this is no product of an ivory tower. They have gathered together an impressive array of topics and the result is, I believe, a book that will soon become one of the standard and well thumbed volumes for anyone seeking to base their work in general practice emergencies on a good foundation of evidence based practice.

Formal training in this area is necessary and should include theoretical teaching and practical experience. The Royal College of General Practitioners has taken an important step by making it a requirement that candidates show their competence at cardiopulmonary resuscitation before they can pass the MRCGP examination. Nevertheless, more skills based courses are needed for established principals. The authors recommend refresher courses to sustain skills on an annual basis. There are frequently gaps in our knowledge about even some of the most potentially life saving activities. This book should go a long way in helping to remedy these gaps. I congratulate the authors on their farsightedness and expertise in producing it.

YVONNE CARTER, MD, FRCGP
Professor of General Practice and Primary Care,
St Bartholomew's
and the Royal London School of Medicine and Dentistry,
Queen Mary and Westfield College, London

Disclaimer

Every effort has been made to ensure that the guidelines and information in this booklet are correct, and represent current and best medical practice. The authors and publishers cannot accept liability for errors arising from the use of this booklet, or for textual errors. The consequences of any medical treatment are entirely the responsibility of the medical practitioner providing it.

"To live through an impossible situation, you don't need the reflexes of a Grand Prix driver, the muscles of a Hercules, the mind of an Einstein. You simply need to know what to do."

The Book of Survival
Anthony Greenbank

Resuscitation

Introduction

Studies looking at the chances of survival around the time of a cardiac arrest have shown that there are several important links in the chain of survival:

1 Early access to the emergency services (**dial 999**)
2 Early basic life support
3 Early defibrillation.

The final step is that of early advanced life support. In general practice the first two steps in this chain can be realistically achieved by all GPs. The third link is feasible although not all GPs do, or wish to, carry a defibrillator. Advanced life support skills are easily learned but it is important that they are kept up to date.

It is vital that all doctors can confidently and reliably perform basic life support.

If you are feeling a bit rusty, there are many ways to refresh/relearn these skills in a friendly and non-threatening environment. You can obtain more information from your local St John's or St Andrew's Ambulance Association, Red Cross Organisation, or the resuscitation training officer at your local hospital.

Basic life support rarely cures the underlying problem—it just buys time until equipment and drugs arrive—so it is essential in all cases that someone has **dialled 999** and ensured that help is on its way.

The following guidelines all conform with those laid down by the Resuscitation Council (UK) and the European Resuscitation Council. We acknowledge their support and permission to reproduce them.

Adult basic life support

Ensure safety of rescuer and victim.

Assess responsiveness: gently shake shoulders and shout "Are you all right?".

If unresponsive

Open **A**irway: remove obvious obstruction; use head tilt and chin lift. If neck injury is suspected use jaw thrust.

Check **B**reathing (max. 10 seconds): look, listen, and feel for chest movements and breath sounds at mouth.

If not **Breathing**

Give two rescue breaths using mouth-to-mouth ventilation.

Check **C**irculation (max. 10 seconds): look for any movement of victim; check carotid pulse.

If pulse present

Continue rescue breathing, recheck every minute for signs of circulation.

If no pulse (or unsure if pulse)

Start chest compressions at 100 times a minute, combined with ventilation (15 compressions to two breaths).

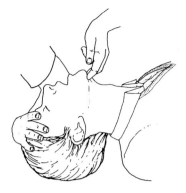

Chin lift in adults. Tilt head with one hand on forehead and lift chin with fingertip(s) under point of victim's chin

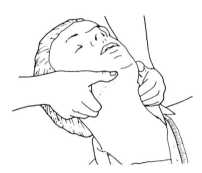

Jaw thrust in adults. Fingers behind angle of lower jaw and press upwards and forwards to lift jaw

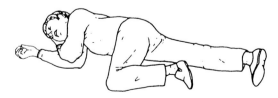

Recovery position in adults. Tilt head to open airway. Use victim's hand under cheek to keep head tilted

Mouth-to-mouth ventilation

- Open **A**irway as above. Occlude nostrils. Ensure a tight seal around the patient's mouth.
- Gently **B**reathe into the patient for about 1.5–2 seconds, ensuring the chest wall rises.

If the chest wall does not move, reassess the airway, adjusting head tilt as necessary. Too vigorous a breath will force air into the stomach (so increasing risk of aspiration, vomiting, etc.).

A disposable *mouth-guard* provides a barrier between you and the victim but does not compromise ventilation. This is just a compact plastic sheet with a filter in the middle. If you possess a *pocket mask*, you can perform mouth-to-mask ventilation instead. Some masks are re-usable and oxygen can be attached if you carry it. There is a one way valve so that you do not breathe in expired air.

Chest compressions

Place the heel of one hand two finger breaths above the xiphisternum and place the other hand on top, interlocking fingers if necessary. Compress the chest to a depth of 4–5 cm, keeping the arms straight and vertically above the chest. The rate is 100 compressions per minute.

Two rescuers: 5 compressions to one breath
One rescuer: 15 compressions to two breaths

Continue cardiopulmonary resuscitation (CPR) until the victim shows signs of life, someone takes over from you, or you are physically exhausted.

Adult advanced life support

The 1997 Resuscitation Guidelines for use in the UK.
These guidelines are based on the ILCOR advisory statements that are being assessed on behalf of the ERC.

The ALS algorithm for the management of cardiac arrest in adults.

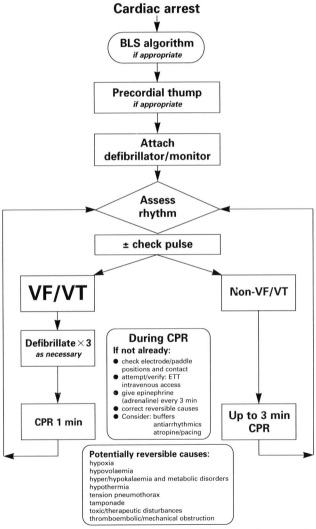

Note that each successive step is based on the assumption that the one before has been unsuccessful.

Paediatric basic life support

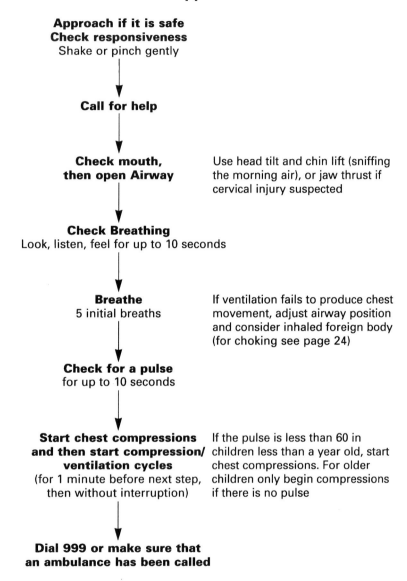

Approach if it is safe
Check responsiveness
Shake or pinch gently

↓

Call for help

↓

Check mouth,
then open Airway

Use head tilt and chin lift (sniffing the morning air), or jaw thrust if cervical injury suspected

↓

Check Breathing
Look, listen, feel for up to 10 seconds

↓

Breathe
5 initial breaths

If ventilation fails to produce chest movement, adjust airway position and consider inhaled foreign body (for choking see page 24)

↓

Check for a pulse
for up to 10 seconds

↓

Start chest compressions
and then start compression/
ventilation cycles
(for 1 minute before next step, then without interruption)

If the pulse is less than 60 in children less than a year old, start chest compressions. For older children only begin compressions if there is no pulse

↓

Dial 999 or make sure that
an ambulance has been called

How to do basic life support in children

	Infant (< 1 year)	Small child (1–8 years)	Larger child
Airway position	Neutral	Sniffing the morning air	Sniffing the morning air
Breathing	Mouth to mouth and nose	Mouth to mouth	Mouth to mouth
Circulation Pulse check	Brachial or femoral	Brachial or carotid	Carotid
Chest compression Landmark	One finger breadth below nipple line	Two finger breadths above xiphoid	Two finger breadths above xiphoid
Technique	Encircling or two fingers	One hand	Two hands
Depth (cm)	1.5–2.5	2.5–3.5	4–5
Ratio of chest compressions to ventilations	5:1	5:1	15:2
Compression rate per minute	100	100	100

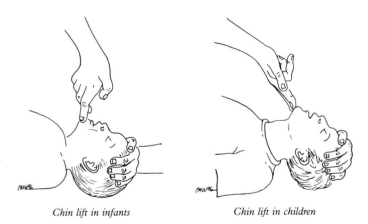

Chin lift in infants   *Chin lift in children*

Jaw thrust in children

Performing artificial ventilation in children

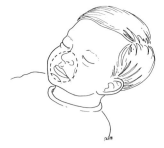

Mouth-to-mouth and mouth-to-nose ventilation in a small child

If you have a pocket mask or bag–valve–mask

- Check that there are no leaks, and that any valves are working.
- If possible use oxygen.
- If the airway is properly opened then using a mask is easy. You can apply a jaw thrust with your fingers while sealing the mask onto the face with your other fingers. Getting someone else to squeeze the bag will free you up to obtain a better seal. You can use a pocket mask upside down to get a better seal on a smaller child.

Performing chest compressions in children

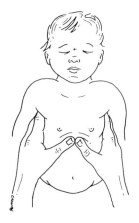

Infant chest compression: hand encircling technique

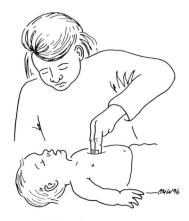

Infant chest compression: two finger technique

General notes on resuscitation

Oxygen

Oxygen is the most important drug at any cardiac arrest—consider carrying a small cylinder.

Epinephrine (adrenaline)

Epinephrine augments basic life support by improving both coronary and cerebral perfusion. Epinephrine is given approximately every 3 minutes (after 10 cycles of basic life support).

Defibrillator

If you possess a defibrillator make sure you can use it quickly and confidently. The sequence of shocks should be given rapidly—check for a pulse after each shock and check rhythm on monitor. Do not restart compression/ventilation between shocks unless the machine takes more than 30 seconds to recharge.

If you do not carry a defibrillator, then continue with basic life support. Ensure that there are no treatable causes of cardiac arrest, such as hypovolaemia, tension pneumothorax, drug overdose, or hypothermia.

Compressions/ventilations

Do not interrupt compressions and ventilations for more than 30 seconds to intubate or gain intravenous access. If necessary abort the attempt and re-try after 10 cycles of basic life support. Drugs (in double dose) can be given down the endotracheal tube if you cannot gain intravenous access.

In most cases, once resuscitation has been started by the doctor it should be continued until the ambulance crew take over. In particular, resuscitation attempts should be prolonged in cases of hypothermia and immersion, and for children. Fixed dilated pupils are not a reliable guide that prolonged resuscitation attempts are futile; they may be the result of hypothermia or drugs (for example, epinephrine).

General management of shock

Many of the conditions covered in this book are associated with shock. Shock is a clinical syndrome resulting from abnormal circulation. This leads to inadequate organ perfusion, poor tissue oxygenation, and insufficient removal of tissue waste products.

The most important thing to bear in mind is that *shock is a progressive condition*. It can be thought of as having three sequential phases: compensated, decompensated, and irreversible. It follows that appropriate and aggressive management should be started as soon as possible. The causes of shock include:

- Hypovolaemia, for example, haemorrhage, dehydration
- Pump failure, for example, myocardial infarction, tension pneumothorax, pulmonary embolism
- Inappropriate distribution of the cardiac output, for example, anaphylaxis, sepsis
- Others, for example, severe anaemia.

In adults

In the early stages there is tachycardia, tachypnoea, sweating, and anxiety. As shock progresses the capillary refill time is prolonged, there is a fall in blood pressure, the patient may become pale and cold to the touch, and there is altered mental state. Remember that in early septic shock the skin may be warm. In young adults hypotension is a dangerous sign, because blood pressure tends to be preserved for longer by sympathetic responses.

In children

In the early stages there is tachycardia and a weak pulse, cool peripheries, and subtle changes such as mild irritability. As shock progresses the tachycardia is more marked, capillary refill time is prolonged, and there is cyanosis with a reduced level of consciousness. Hypotension is a late and sinister sign, as is a skin that is pale and cold to the touch.

To assess capillary refill time, simply compress a fingernail, and see how long it takes for the pink colour to return when released. Capillary refill time is prolonged if it is longer than two seconds.

The ABC of treating shock

Airway and Breathing

Is the airway clear? If not use the techniques described in the basic life support sections. If there has been trauma you should preferentially use the jaw thrust manoeuvre to open the airway and you must protect the cervical spine. Give the highest concentration of oxygen you can.

Circulation

Establish intravenous access. Use the largest cannula you can, in the largest and most accessible vein.

- In adults give Hartmann's solution as indicated. Generally it is safe to start with 500 ml–1 litre on the way to hospital. You can give more fluids if the response is poor or inadequate. Remember to be cautious in the presence of heart failure or head injury. If you suspect an abdominal aortic aneurysm, aim for a systolic blood pressure of no more than 100 mm Hg.
- In children start with Hartmann's solution 20 ml/kg as a bolus, giving further boluses of 10–20 ml/kg as clinically indicated.

    In children under six years of age the technique of intraosseous infusion is becoming more widespread and is being used in the community. It is used if intravenous access cannot be established. It is described in detail on page 84.

Other measures

Lie the patient as flat as possible with the legs raised, or in the recovery position if unconscious (unless there has been trauma). Keep the patient warm. Check the temperature and blood glucose.

Adult medical emergencies

Choking in adults

Ensure an ambulance is on the way. Remove the obstruction if visible.

Patient able to breathe and conscious

Encourage coughing and give oxygen if you carry it.

Patient unable to breathe—completely obstructed airway

If conscious

Up to five *backslaps* (between the shoulder blades with the heel of the hand). If unsuccessful, up to five *abdominal thrusts* (Heimlich manoeuvre; see page 78). Direct the thrusts upwards towards the diaphragm.

Recheck in the mouth—you may have dislodged the obstruction. If not continue with backslaps and abdominal thrusts.

If unconscious

Try *finger sweeps* to remove the obstruction. If unsuccessful, then five *abdominal thrusts* with the patient lying flat on the floor. If still unsuccessful then use *chest compressions* (see page 4). Try to ventilate at least every minute.

Continue above manoeuvres until obstruction is relieved. If you are still unsuccessful, then consider needle cricothyroidotomy (see page 82).

For choking in children, see page 24.

Anaphylaxis in adults

Suspect anaphylaxis as a cause for sudden collapse even if there is no previous history of allergy. Symptoms and signs vary in severity and may include rash (erythema, urticaria, or flushing), bronchospasm, pulmonary oedema, tachycardia, hypotension, diarrhoea and vomiting, and angio-oedema.

Call an ambulance.

Airway

- Ensure it is clear and give oxygen if you carry it
- Give *epinephrine 0.5–1 mg i.m.*
  (0.5–1.0 ml of 1:1000 *or* 5–10 ml of 1:10 000)
- Repeat *epinephrine* every 5–10 minutes as required.

Breathing

- Start artificial ventilation if necessary
- Assess for bronchospasm.

Circulation

- If no palpable pulse start cardiac compressions.

Secure intravenous access and give intravenous fluids if hypotensive. Start with 500 ml of Hartmann's. Intravenous epinephrine is rarely required unless severely hypotensive, in which case give 0.5 mg (0.5 ml of 1:1000 or 5 ml of 1:10 000) by slow injection.

Other treatments

- *Antihistamines*—chlorpheniramine 10 mg i.v. (over 1 min) especially if angio-oedema (dilute with patient's blood before use).
- *Steroids*—hydrocortisone 200 mg i.v. especially if bronchospasm.
- *Salbutamol*—5 mg by nebuliser if bronchospasm.

All cases of anaphylaxis require observation and possibly further treatment, so refer to hospital. Symptoms may recur.

Acute asthma in adults

Patients still die in the UK from acute asthmatic attacks. Many of these deaths are avoidable. When faced with an asthmatic patient who complains of increasing wheeze or breathlessness, first decide whether the attack is mild, severe, or life threatening. The guidelines below are based on those of the British Thoracic Society.

Mild/moderate attack

The patient may be breathless but not distressed, with a peak flow of 50–70% of expected. Treatment is to increase the β agonist, double the inhaled steroids, and consider oral steroids (prednisolone 30–60 mg). Review should be arranged to obtain an overview of the patient's asthma.

Severe attack

The patient may be too wheezy to complete sentences (but equally may not be distressed), and has peak flow of <50% of expected, respiration of > 25/min, and pulse > 110/min.

> Give high flow oxygen and nebulised salbutamol 5 mg/terbutaline 10 mg (if possible drive the nebuliser with oxygen)
> or
> 10–40 puffs β agonist from inhaler via spacer device (one puff at a time)
> *and*
> prednisolone 30–60 mg orally
> *and/or*
> hydrocortisone 200 mg i.v.
> ↓
> *Assess after 15 min*
> ↓
> If poor response admit
> or
> If good response and peak flow >50% of expected, *still admit if you have doubts*, or step up treatment plus oral dose of steroids

Life threatening asthma

The patient will be exhausted and confused, or may even be comatose with peak flow of less than 33% of expected, bradycardia or hypotension, silent chest, or cyanosis.

Give high flow oxygen, and nebulised salbutamol 5 mg/terbutaline 10 mg (if possible drive the nebuliser with oxygen)

or

10–40 puffs β-agonist from inhaler via spacer device (one puff at a time)

and

prednisolone 30–60 mg orally

and/or

hydrocortisone 200 mg i.v.

and

ipratropium 0.5 mg nebule
↓
ADMIT

Patients with life threatening asthma may not appear distressed and may not have all of the clinical signs detailed above. The presence of **any** *of these clinical signs should alert the doctor.*

The following factors should reduce the threshold for admission:

- Night time waking or morning exacerbations
- Seen in the afternoon or early evening
- Recent hospital admission
- Past history of severe attacks, especially of rapid onset
- Poor social support or understanding of own condition.

15

Management of acute myocardial infarction

If possible arrange to meet the emergency ambulance at the patient's home, that is, **Dial 999**. Most deaths are from ventricular fibrillation, usually within the first hour.

Airway and Breathing

Give oxygen if available.

Circulation

Establish intravenous access if possible.

Give sublingual nitrate

If the patient has cardiac chest pain, unless he has already received adequate doses, or unless there is hypotension (systolic BP <90 mm Hg). GTN (glyceryl trinitrate) can precipitate sudden hypotension.

Give intravenous opiates

Use diamorphine (2.5–5 mg) or morphine sulphate (5–10 mg) in increments, along with metoclopramide 10 mg. Avoid intramuscular administration if at all possible because this interferes with cardiac enzyme assays, and can result in haematoma formation if thrombolysis is used in hospital.

Aspirin

This is recommended if the patient has not had any in the preceding 24 hours. In this case give 150 mg to chew. Contraindications are: known hypersensitivity, bleeding peptic ulcer, blood dyscrasia, known hepatic disease.

- Stay with the patient until the ambulance arrives.
- You should be prepared to deal with the arrhythmias that go with myocardial infarction, especially ventricular fibrillation.

Thrombolysis

The ideal target is that patients will receive thrombolysis within 60 min, and certainly within 90 min, of their symptom onset. If your practice is some distance from the hospital, consider whether you should be giving thrombolysis at home. You should be doing this within local protocols, and with the support of your local cardiology unit. We do not therefore give doses/protocols, etc., but will leave room for these if relevant to your particular set up.

Acute pulmonary oedema

Has there been a myocardial infarction? If it seems likely, arrange to meet the emergency ambulance at the patient's house, that is, **Dial 999**.

Airway and Breathing

Sit the patient up. Give high flow oxygen if available.

Circulation

Establish intravenous access if possible.

Give diuretic

Frusemide is the most common drug (dose: 40–80 mg i.v. slowly), or bumetanide can be used (dose: 1–2 mg i.v.).

Give intravenous opiates

Use diamorphine (2.5–5 mg) or morphine sulphate (5–10 mg) in increments, along with metoclopramide 10 mg.

Give sublingual nitrate

Unless the patient is hypotensive (systolic BP < 90 mm Hg) or has had adequate doses already.

Acute pulmonary embolism

The pre-hospital management of this condition is based on giving high flow oxygen, and establishing intravenous access to give opiates such as diamorphine. Avoid giving intramuscular analgesia because this may lead to haematoma formation if the patient is thrombolysed in hospital.

Seizures in adults

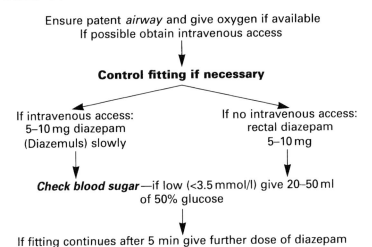

Ensure patent *airway* and give oxygen if available
If possible obtain intravenous access

Control fitting if necessary

If intravenous access:
5–10 mg diazepam
(Diazemuls) slowly

If no intravenous access:
rectal diazepam
5–10 mg

Check blood sugar—if low (<3.5 mmol/l) give 20–50 ml
of 50% glucose

If fitting continues after 5 min give further dose of diazepam

Remember fitting may be secondary to other pathology, for example, head injury, drug overdose, infection, metabolic imbalance, tumours, etc.

Refer to hospital if

- First fits, prolonged or uncontrollable fits
- Atypical fits for that patient or increase in frequency
- Suspicion of other underlying pathology
- No social support to observe during post-ictal period.

19

Coma in adults

First ask yourself: *is this patient unconscious?*

Easy ways of assessing conscious level are using either the **AVPU** system or the Glasgow Coma Score.

A **A**lert
V responds to **V**ocal stimuli
P responds to **P**ainful stimuli
U **U**nresponsive to any stimuli.

The Glasgow Coma Score is assessed on the motor verbal and eye opening responses with a maximum score of 15. It takes longer to assess and is hard to remember at times of crisis so is not as useful in an emergency. Any score of 8 or less is defined as unconscious.

Eye opening

4 opens eyes spontaneously
3 opens eyes to verbal stimuli
2 opens eyes to painful stimuli
1 does not open eyes

Motor response

6 obeys commands
5 localises pain
4 flexion withdrawal of limb to pain
3 abnormal (decerebrate) flexion of limb to pain
2 extension to pain
1 no response

Verbal response

5 alert and orientated
4 confused
3 inappropriate speech
2 incomprehensible sounds, for example, moans
1 no verbal response

There are multiple aetiologies for the unconscious patient. Most will not resolve spontaneously with out-of-hospital treatment.

Ensure the ambulance is on its way.

Airway

- Is it clear? Remove any foreign bodies/vomit
- Administer oxygen if you carry it
- If you suspect head injury, immobilise the cervical spine as far as possible (see page 76). Use a jaw thrust rather than a head tilt to open the airway.

Breathing

- Check respiratory rate and pattern
- If necessary supplement with mouth-to-mouth or bag–valve–mask ventilation.

Circulation

- Check pulse and BP
- If no output start cardiac compression
- Obtain intravenous access and give intravenous fluids if hypotensive.

Check blood sugar (BM stix)

- If <3.5 mmol/l give 20–50 ml of 50% glucose i.v.

Check pupils

- If pinpoint consider opiate overdose. Give naloxone 100–200 μg i.v. if available. Repeat as needed. Remember that naloxone has a shorter half life than most opiates, so when the naloxone wears off there may be a late collapse.

Brief examination for possible cause of unconsciousness; in particular consider (and treat if possible): infection, overdose or poisoning, hypo- or hyperglycaemia, hypoxia, post-ictal state, cerebrovascular accident, subarachnoid haemorrhage, trauma, and hypothermia. Do not induce emesis in an unconscious patient with suspected poisoning—you may seriously compromise the airway.

Paediatric medical emergencies

Quick assessment of the sick child

Airway and Breathing

- Is the airway clear?
- Work of breathing—grunting, nasal flaring, recession, or indrawing
- Respiratory rate
- Auscultation
- Is there cyanosis?

Circulation

- Heart rate
- Pulse volume—is it thready, easily felt, etc.?
- Capillary refill time: to assess this compress a fingernail, and see how long it takes for the pink colour to return when released; it should be less than two seconds
- Skin temperature.

Disability:

- Posture and tone—is the child floppy, playful, etc.?
- Pupillary reactions
- Mental status—the **AVPU** scale:

A **A**lert
V responds to **V**erbal stimuli
P responds to **P**ainful stimuli
U **U**nresponsive

If the child is sick **Dial 999**. It is better to call for help early. If the child needs to be in hospital the options are to "scoop and run", or "stay and stabilise". It is always worth considering what can be done to stabilise the child before transporting.

Useful paediatric data

Normal values for respiratory and heart rates

Age (years)	Respiratory rate (/min)	Heart rate (/min)
<1	30–40	110–160
2–5	20–30	95–140
5–12	15–20	80–120
>12	12–16	60–100

Weight chart, and how much fluid to give in shock

Age	Approximate weight (kg)	Fluid bolus in shock (ml)
3 months	6	120
6 months	8	160
9 months	9	180
1 year	10	200
2 years	12	240
6 years	20	400
10 years	30	600
12 years	40	800
14 years	50	1000

The figures are based on the current growth charts, at the 50th centile. They are only approximate. The fluid bolus is calculated on the basis of 20 ml/kg.

The weight in kg can also be quickly estimated as:

2 (age + 4) in children over 1 year.

The fluid can be given as a bolus using a syringe, or as a rapid intravenous infusion. In hospital colloids such as human albumin tend to be used in shock, but in the pre-hospital environment it is acceptable to use an isotonic non-glucose containing solution such as Hartmann's solution. Avoid using 5% dextrose in children.

Choking in children (see also pages 76 and 77)

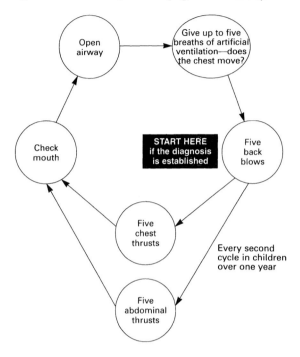

Do not perform blind finger sweeps.

Back blows are delivered between the shoulder blades. The child's head should be lower than his abdomen.

Chest thrusts are similar to chest compressions except they are more vigorous, but with a slower rhythm. They should be performed at a rate of one every three seconds. Lie the child on his back, if possible head down along the knee.

Abdominal thrusts can be performed in children over a year of age. Use Heimlich's manoeuvre in conscious children or lay the unconscious child on his or her back. Direct the thrusts upwards towards the diaphragm.

Continue the circuits until the foreign body is cleared.

(Cricothyroidotomy is described in the Practical procedures section, page 82.)

Anaphylactic shock in children

- Stop the allergen if known.
- Assess **A**irway, **B**reathing, and **C**irculation. If there is respiratory or cardiac arrest, commence basic life support (page 6). **Dial 999**.
- Give high flow oxygen if available.

Epinephrine (adrenaline)

This is the mainstay of treatment. The dose is 10 µg/kg i.m. *Repeat the dose every 10 min*, if there is no improvement or deterioration. This dose can be given intravenously if there is cardiac arrest.

Age (years)	Dose of i.m. epinephrine 1:1000 (ml)
<1	0.05
1	0.1
2	0.2
3–4	0.3
5	0.4
6–12	0.5
Adult	0.5–1.0

These doses are for children of average weight. Halve the doses in underweight children. To give the smallest doses it may be best to dilute the epinephrine in saline, in which case you will need to multiply up the volumes given in the table.

If there is airway obstruction with stridor, you can in addition give the child nebulised epinephrine at a dose of 5 ml of 1:1000. If you don't have that much epinephrine to hand, dilute what you have up to 5 ml, using 0.9% saline.

Additional measures

1 Give fluids if there is shock. Use a 20 ml/kg bolus, repeated if necessary.
2 Give nebulised salbutamol if the patient is wheezy (dose: 5 mg in children over two years, halved in children under two years). If the wheeze continues, repeat the nebuliser as required, and give hydrocortisone in a dose of 4 mg/kg i.v.
3 If there is a rash give an oral antihistamine. Also consider oral prednisolone at a dose of 1–2 mg/kg, rounded to the nearest 5 mg, maximum dose 40 mg.

Acute severe asthma in children

Judging the severity

The first task when faced with a child with acute asthma is to assess the severity. You may find this table helpful.

	Mild/moderate	Severe	Life threatening
Level of consciousness	Normal	Altered	Altered
Exhaustion	Nil ——————————————➤ Present		
Cyanosis	Nil ——————————————➤ Present		
Wheeze	Yes	Yes	Silent chest
Retraction	Absent/mild	Present	Obvious
Accessory muscle use	Absent	Present	Obvious
Palpable pulsus paradoxus	No ——————————————➤ Yes		
Initial peak flow (% predicted or usual)	>50–60	<50	<33
Behaviour	Active	Inactive	Sedated

Several factors should also be considered when judging the medical response:

- Previous pattern of response to trigger factors
- Previous admission to ICU with asthma
- Previous requirement for intravenous therapy
- Frequent hospital attendances/admissions
- Currently using oral steroids
- Recent hospital discharge
- Social factors such as availability of a telephone, understanding of severity.

In general, don't be afraid to treat asthma aggressively. This condition can deteriorate rapidly. If you do not admit the child, you will need to make arrangements for reassessment.

Management of severe asthma

Dial 999
↓
Give oxygen if available, high flow, via face mask
↓
Salbutamol 5 mg or terbutaline 10 mg via nebuliser

(Halve these doses in children under two years)
↓
Oral prednisolone 2 mg/kg (max. 40 mg) rounded to the nearest 5 mg
|
If life threatening features are present:
↓
Give salbutamol/terbutaline nebulisers as frequently as necessary while effecting transfer
↓
Add ipratropium 0·25 mg to the nebuliser

(This cannot be repeated more than 6 hourly)

The nebuliser should be oxygen driven if possible. Make up the volume to about 4 ml using 0·9% saline (not water for injection). Oxygen should be continued for at least 15 min after the drug is delivered.

If you haven't got a nebuliser use a spacer device instead (see the Hints section on page 75).

These guidelines are based on the recommendations of the British Thoracic Society.

Septic shock in children

Dial 999
↓
Airway—ensure this is clear

Breathing—give oxygen if available

Circulation—try to obtain intravenous access if the child
needs urgent treatment

Give 20 ml/kg fluid boluses as required
↓
Exclude hypoglycaemia

If glucose <3 mmol/l give 10% glucose 5 ml/kg i.v. or 50%
glucose 1–2 ml/kg i.v. The last is irritant to young veins

(You can also use glucagon 0·5–1·0 unit i.m., s.c., or i.v., or if
the child is sufficiently awake Hypostop gel is a further
alternative)
↓
● If you suspect meningococcal disease—give
benzylpenicillin i.v. or i.m.

Benzylpenicillin dose:

Age < 1 year use 300 mg

Age 1–10 years use 600 mg

Age > 10 years use 1200 mg

Do not worry about interfering with hospital tests, although
you can take a throat swab first and send it in with the
patient

● In severe sepsis or suspected meningococcal disease in
the presence of penicillin allergy—alternative broad
spectrum antibiotics include:

Cefotaxime: dose is 100 mg/kg i.v. or i.m. (small volume)

Ceftriaxone: dose is 50 mg/kg i.v. or i.m. (larger volume)

Stridor in children

The first task when seeing a child with stridor is to make a provisional diagnosis, because this will influence the management significantly. It is vital to differentiate croup from epiglottitis, and to differentiate both of these from other causes.

Differentiating croup from epiglottitis

Feature	Croup	Epiglottitis
Aetiology	Mostly parainfluenza virus	*Haemophilus influenzae* b
Onset	Over days	Over hours
Preceding coryza	Yes	No
Cough	Severe, barking	Absent or slight
Able to drink?	Yes	No
Drooling?	No	Yes
Appearance	Unwell	Toxic and ill
Temperature	< 38·5°C	> 38·5°C
Stridor	Harsh, rasping	Soft
Voice	Hoarse	Reluctant to speak, muffled
Wheeze?	Often present	No
Child's posture	Irritable, active	Sitting forward, neck extended

Remember atypical cases may occur.

Other causes

There are other causes of stridor, including: laryngeal foreign body, diphtheria, retropharyngeal abscess, infectious mononucleosis, angioneurotic oedema, hot gas inhalation, laryngomalacia, congenital deformities.

Acute epiglottitis

If you have made this diagnosis, **Dial 999**

↓

Do not do anything else unless the patient obstructs his airway:

—calm and reassure

—nurse upright

—never leave alone

Do not examine the throat

↓

If the patient obstructs his or her airway

Either intubate, which can be difficult, or perform a cricothyroidotomy

(see Practical procedures, page 82)

Many GPs would accompany such a child to the hospital in the ambulance, if circumstances permit.

Croup

The basic signs to look for to assess the severity of croup are shown in the table.

Sign	Less severe $\longrightarrow$	More severe
Stridor	None	At rest, obvious
Cyanosis	None	Obvious
Recession	None	Present
Air entry	Good	Poor
Respiration	Normal	Tachypnoeic
Pulse	Normal	Tachycardic

Any assessment of severity and need for admission are tempered by social circumstances, access to a telephone and a car, availability of medical review, and the child's medical history.

Treatment of severe croup

Dial 999

General measures such as reassurance and plenty of fluids apply in severe croup as for milder forms. Steam inhalation probably has no medical benefit, but distracts the carers and ensures their presence at the child's side.

Give oxygen, if available, in a high concentration.

Nebulised epinephrine (adrenaline): this is useful if you are trying to buy time before the child gets to hospital. Epinephrine can be given through a nebuliser in a dose of 0·5 ml/kg of 1:1000, up to a maximum of 5 ml. Make up smaller doses to 5 ml with saline, not water. Stop the nebuliser if the child's pulse exceeds 180/min. The improvement is transient and there is a rebound effect.

Steroids may be used by the hospital team.

Seizures in children

Airway: Is it clear?
Breathing: Give high flow oxygen
if available

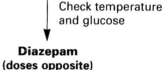

Check temperature
and glucose

Be thinking:

*Is it a seizure? (and not a
rigor, etc.)*

Does it need treatment?

What is the cause?

Febrile
Change of medication
Acute cerebral trauma
Epilepsy
Meningitis or encephalitis
Poisoning
Metabolic disorder
Space occupying lesion
Hypoxia

**Diazepam
(doses opposite)**

If febrile, rectal paracetamol
and cooling manoeuvres such as
removal of clothing, electric fan

Paracetamol doses:
1–5 years: 125–250 mg rectally
6–12 years: 250–500 mg rectally

If still fitting after
5 min

**Diazepam
(doses opposite)**

If the child is still fitting after all this, all
you can do is place him in the recovery
position, maintain airway and breathing,
and wait for the ambulance

Drug dosages and use

Diazepam

Rectal: Age < 1 year use 2·5 mg
          Age 1–3 years use 5 mg
          Age > 3 years use 10 mg

The initial diazepam dose should terminate seizure activity within 5 min. The effect lasts a maximum of 1 hour. It is a respiratory depressant, and a sedative, and can cause hypotension in young infants.

In hypoglycaemia (blood sugar <3 mmol)

Use glucose if you can get intravenous access, glucagon if you cannot.

Glucose dose

5 ml/kg of 10% glucose or 1–2 ml/kg of 50% glucose solution i.v. 50% glucose is highly irritant to veins. Flush through thoroughly.

Glucagon dose

0·5–1·0 unit s.c., i.m., or i.v. This should work within 15 min and, if it doesn't, you are left with trying to gain intravenous access again to give glucose.

If you suspect meningococcal disease

Give benzylpenicillin i.v. or i.m.

Benzylpenicillin dose:

         Age < 1 year use 300 mg
         Age 1–10 years use 600 mg
         Age > 10 years use 1200 mg

Do not worry about interfering with hospital tests, although you can take a throat swab first and send it in with the patient.

In severe sepsis or suspected meningococcal disease in the presence of penicillin allergy

Alternative broad spectrum antibiotics include:

Cefotaxime: dose is 100 mg/kg i.v. or i.m. (small volume)
Ceftriaxone: dose is 50 mg/kg i.v. or i.m. (larger volume)

Coma in children

Coma in children is always an emergency—**Dial 999**

Airway: Is the airway clear?

If there is a history of trauma stabilise the cervical spine

Breathing: Give high flow oxygen if available

Assist ventilation if necessary

Circulation: You may need to try and gain intravenous access
↓
Exclude hypoglycaemia

If glucose < 3 mmol/l give 10% glucose 5 ml/kg i.v. or 50% glucose 1–2 ml/kg i.v. The last is irritant to young veins

You can also use glucagon 0·5–1·0 unit i.m., s.c., or i.v.

The counsel of perfection is to take 10 ml clotted blood and send it in with the child for diagnostic studies
↓
Rapid general physical assessment and history looking for causes
↓
If there is hypovolaemic or septic shock, you should consider starting treatment. Use the relevant sections

Causes of coma in children

Hypoxia, seizures, trauma, sepsis, poisons, metabolic causes, hypertension, space occupying lesions, intussusception.

What to do at a road traffic accident

It is not uncommon for GPs to come across road accidents, and it is possible that you will be asked to attend one. This chapter offers some guidance as to what to do if faced with such a situation.

Getting there and parking safely

If you are asked to attend an accident, drive quickly but safely and within the law. You have no right to exceed the speed limit or to ignore road signs and traffic lights. Use dipped headlights and a green beacon if you have one. It may be safer to arrange a police vehicle to take you to the scene. Don't forget to ensure that the Ambulance Service and Police have been called.

Park safely. If the accident scene is exposed to oncoming traffic, park so that your car will protect you and the scene. Leave your hazard lights on, and if available use a warning triangle. Leave your keys in the ignition in case the Police need to move your car later. Wear high visibility clothing, if possible, and put on some gloves. Identify yourself to the ambulance personnel.

Your personal safety is paramount.

Assessment

Have a quick look at any vehicle damage. It will give you an idea of the nature of the impact and likely injuries. Ensure that it is safe to approach.

If you are on your own, *take command*. Ask any helpers to stop or direct the traffic, and check that the emergency services have been called. Use the following ETHANE mnenomic to gather the details needed by ambulance control:

E   Exact location
T   Type of incident
H   Hazards (check HAZCHEM signs on any tankers involved)
A   Access for emergency services
N   Number of casualties
E   Emergency services present and those still needed

If any car engines are running, turn them off.

Now you can go on to triage.

Road traffic accident

Triage

Triage means "to sort". Make a rapid appraisal of who needs what, and in what order. There are unlikely to be more than one or two seriously injured people, but if there are then triage according to the following priorities

- Check the **A**irway and **B**reathing of all casualties
- Return to the seriously injured to deal with **C**irculatory problems.

Delegate bystanders to look after and comfort the less seriously injured, asking them to report any changes in condition. Use simple clear instructions like "I want you to sit with him, hold his hand, and talk to him, but let me know if he becomes unconscious".

Remember your ABC

In pre-hospital trauma care you are looking after the basics:

Airway with control of the cervical spine
Breathing
Circulation

If time permits you can think about other injuries. Do not waste time at the scene unless you believe your actions will improve outcome or suffering—transport the patients to hospital as soon as it is safe to do so.

Airway

An open airway is essential. Beware unconscious patients sitting upright, with the head slumped—occluding the airway. Beware loose dentures, but leave well fitted ones in place. Open the airway using the the "jaw thrust" manoeuvre described on page 3. This helps protect the cervical spine.

Cervical spine control is a part of airway management. Details are given on page 76.

36

If a jaw thrust has not succeeded in clearing the airway, try a gentle finger sweep. If this is unsuccessful you will need to do more. The sequence is as follows:

1 Oropharyngeal airway: this cannot be used in conscious patients or those with a gag reflex. Select an airway that corresponds in length to the distance between the incisor teeth and the angle of the jaw (usually sizes 2, 3, and 4). In adults insert upside down—concave side upwards—then rotate through 180° once the tongue is passed. In children insert the right way up—gently.
2 Nasopharyngeal airway: if you have one and know how to use it, or if the ambulance crew carry some, this is useful next. It is used to protect the airway in patients who cannot tolerate an oropharyngeal airway.
3 Intubation: only attempt this if you know what you are doing.
4 In the event of an obstructed upper airway you may have no choice but to attempt a needle circothyroidotomy. The technique is described on page 82. It is not easy to do, but may save a life.

Breathing

LOOK for bruising or unequal chest wall movement. Count the respiratory rate. Look for sucking chest wounds.

FEEL for tracheal position, chest wall tenderness, and surgical emphysema

LISTEN to the air entry if you can hear anything above all the noise—and give oxygen in the highest available concentration

There are two treatable and life threatening conditions to look for:

• Tension pneumothorax: the casualty has respiratory distress, a trachea deviated away from the problem, and a resonant chest on the side of the problem. You may be able to hear reduced air entry over the pneumothorax. The treatment is needle thoracocentesis, described on page 80. This procedure can save a life.
• Sucking chest wound: simply cover the wound with a gauze square, taped down on three sides. Leave the fourth side untaped to act as a one way valve.

Circulation

LOOK for signs of external blood loss and pallor. The capillary refill time is less than two seconds in well perfused patients. Simply compress a fingernail, and see how long it takes for the pink colour to return when released. A prolonged capillary refill time is a sign of severe shock.

FEEL the pulse and take a blood pressure if you can. A rough guide is:

- Palpable radial pulse implies systolic BP > 90 mm Hg
- Palpable femoral pulse implies systolic BP > 70 mm Hg
- Palpable carotid pulse implies systolic BP > 60 mm Hg.

Remember that in children and young adults hypotension and poor perfusion are late signs of shock—if there is a tachycardia in these groups suspect significant blood loss.

- Stop external bleeding with pressure dressings and elevation.
- Establish venous access with the largest cannula you can, and in the largest and most accessible vein you can get at. In children, intraosseous needles are increasingly used if venous access cannot be obtained and is needed urgently (see page 84). If the hospital is within 20 minutes of travel time, and the patient is not trapped, it may be better to scoop-and-run—attempting venous access en route.
- Give fluids. It is acceptable to give 1 litre of Hartmann's solution (or 20 ml/kg in children), increasing to 2 litres if there is hypotension. If there is an isolated head or chest injury, with no evidence of shock, start fluids more cautiously.

Disability

This is best assessed using the AVPU score, and pupillary responses:

A **A**lert
V responds to **V**erbal commands
P responds to **P**ain
U **U**nresponsive

Be alert to changes in conscious level.

Analgesia

Pain control is a high priority. Simple reassurance, using first names, and engaging in simple conversation have an important role.

Nitrous oxide is acceptable and may be used unless there is a pneumothorax or open skull fracture.

Diamorphine is the best opiate to use. Give metoclopramide 10 mg i.v. first, and then diamorphine i.v. in 1 mg aliquots until pain is controlled. Diluting the diamorphine in 10 ml water aids titration. You should have naloxone available when giving diamorphine in this way.

Make a note of what drugs you use and when. A good idea is to write drug and fluid doses on the casualty's forehead with an indelible marker. Make sure the ambulance crew know what you have given if you are not travelling to hospital with the patient.

Entrapment

Extricating a trapped patient can be a long and difficult task, and good teamwork with the ambulance and fire crews is essential. Stick to the **ABC**s and ensure analgesia is adequate, because this will help the other members of the team. If there is likely to be a significant delay, consider calling out a hospital team who carry equipment and blood, may be able to give more powerful anaesthesia, and can sometimes perform amputations. A local BASICS doctor may also be available to help.

Transport to hospital

Consider going to hospital with the patient. Ask the Police if they will bring your car along for you. Once in A&E you can hand over to the hospital team, and perhaps have a chat with the ambulance crew and senior A&E staff about how things went. It is also a good chance to replenish your stocks.

Special situations

Burns

Airway

Suspect an inhalational injury if there are burns or soot around or in the mouth or nose, singed nasal hairs, stridor, or wheeze. Give oxygen if you carry it and arrange *urgent* transfer to hospital.

Breathing

Inhalational injury and/or toxic fume exposure increases the risk of pulmonary oedema. A full thickness burn to the chest can reduce chest wall movement especially if circumferential.

Support breathing by mask or other ventilation as necessary. Avoid fluid overload if you suspect significant lung damage.

Circulation

A burns patient can lose large amounts of fluid and can easily become hypovolaemic.

Site at least one intravenous cannula, if possible, through non-burnt skin. Give fluids, for example, Hartmann's solution. In an adult start with 1 litre and in a child 20 ml/kg.

Analgesia

Burns are extremely painful. Intravenous opiates are the best, titrating the amount in small increments. Otherwise use an intramuscular bolus, for example, morphine i.m.:

Adult   5–10 mg
Infant <1 year 0·1 mg/kg
Child > 1 year 0·2 mg/kg

Other injuries

Patients may have other injuries—especially if they have jumped from a height to escape a burning building, for example, spinal, limb, or head injuries. **A**irway, **B**reathing, and **C**irculation still take priority. If there is a reduced conscious level, treat hypoxia and hypovolaemia first before assuming it is the result of a head injury. Beware of coincidental pathology—psychiatric, alcoholic, and epileptic patients are all at increased risk of burn injury.

Thickness of burns

- Superficial: erythema or blistered, painful
- Partial thickness: blistered (often with white base), may have reduced sensation
- Full thickness: leathery, white or charred, painless, numb.

Ensure all but very superficial burns are reassessed at 36–48 hours as apparent thickness may change. Refer if necessary.

Treatment

Cool the burn with water or damp cloths for about 10 minutes if this has not already been done, but do not make the patient hypothermic. Then cover with a dressing—cling film is the best or clean linen. Burns are tetanus prone wounds—ensure the patient is up to date with his or her boosters. There is no need to give prophylactic antibiotics.

Refer to hospital

- All full thickness burns bigger than a 10p coin.
- Any burn of more than a few per cent. The area of the patient's hand is approximately equal to 1% of body surface area.
- Burns of special areas such as eyelids, face, neck, hands, and perineum, or across joints.

Special situations

Electrocution

Most importantly *ensure your own safety.*

Ensure all electricity is turned off before you approach the casualty. High voltage (industrial currents) can arc over several feet so you can still be at risk even if you are not in direct contact with the current source.

Most domestic and industrial electricity is AC (domestic 240 V, commercial 415 V and higher); lightning is DC.

Airway and Breathing

Electric current may cause paralysis of respiratory muscles which can persist for 30 minutes or longer, so resuscitation may need to be prolonged.

Circulation

Treat arrhythmias, cardiac arrest, and hypovolaemia (secondary to burns), according to standard protocols.

AC voltage commonly causes ventricular fibrillation.

DC voltage may cause asystole.

Referral

All except the most minor of shocks should be referred to hospital for a period of observation and ECG monitoring, especially for those with a cardiac history. Beware of the possibility of other injuries, for example, fractures secondary to a fall, or electrical or flame burns.

Hanging

A special consideration is the *risk of cervical spine injury*, even though many deaths resulting from hanging are secondary to asphyxia and hypoxia rather than the classic hangman's fracture. If the patient has not already been cut down, obtain help and carry him or her to the ground supporting the head and neck as you do so.

- *Immobilise the neck*: try to ensure it is neither flexed nor hyperextended, and do not pull on the neck as there is risk of further damage (see page 76 for immobilisation techniques).
- Open the airway using a *jaw thrust or chin lift* manoeuvre. Do not use head tilt (see page 3).
- Give *oxygen* if you carry it.
- Start *basic life support* (and advanced life support) as necessary according to the standard protocols.
- Be aware of the possibility of *other injuries* or pathology— particularly an overdose or attempt at other self harm.

Ensure that you have *documented* all the procedures and actions you performed. There will almost always be some form of police enquiry into the case. Once the patient is safely on his or her way to hospital, spend a few minutes writing everything down that you can remember (including details of the initial scene), while it is still clear in your mind.

Special situations

Near drowning

There is no difference in the management of near drowning in salt or fresh water.

Dial 999—ensure help is on its way.

Ensure your own safety. If removing the victim from water, do so with the patient horizontal or slightly head down.

Attempt to resuscitate all patients

Coexistent hypothermia affords some measure of protection against hypoxic brain damage, especially in children. Long term survival has been reported after submersion for up to an hour.

Airway and Breathing

If there is a suspicion of neck injury (for example, after diving into shallow water), use a jaw thrust not a head tilt to open the airway. Don't forget to remove seaweed and other debris. Start ventilation if needed (see page 4).

Circulation

Hypothermia may make the chest wall stiffer than normal and it also increases the risk of arrhythmias; these are treated according to standard protocols.

Beware of extreme bradycardia: feel for a pulse for more than 10 seconds if necessary. There may be an apparent hypovolaemia (with circulating fluid pushed into the tissues) so intravenous fluids may be required.

Hypothermia

This is defined as a core temperature below 35°C. You may need a low reading thermometer to confirm this. Risk factors include exposure to cold water, wet conditions, or wind for prolonged periods, immobility (especially in elderly people), and children (as a result of their relatively large surface area).

You must attempt resuscitation in all cases—*you are not dead until you are warm and dead.*

Hypothermia protects vital organs to a certain extent. Dilated pupils occur with hypotension, hypoglycaemia, and some drugs, so fixed dilated pupils are not a contraindication to resuscitation.

As body temperature falls, there is a recognised progression of arrhythmias. This is usually sinus bradycardia, atrial fibrillation, ventricular fibrillation, and then asystole.

Resuscitation protocols are the same (see page 5).

If extreme bradycardia, you may need to feel for a pulse for at least one minute. The chest wall may be very stiff so compress at a slower rate to overcome the increased resistance.

Ventricular fibrillation may not respond to cardioversion once the body temperature falls below 30°C so continue basic life support and try to rewarm.

Vigorous cardiopulmonary resuscitation, attempts to intubate, and other mechanical disturbance may precipitate ventricular fibrillation so try to move the patient as little as possible. Administration of oxygen reduces this risk.

Rewarming

Remove cold and wet clothing and wrap in dry blankets or whatever is available. If outside, try to protect from cold winds, etc. Arrange urgent transfer to hospital for more active rewarming.

Gynaecological emergencies

Vaginal bleeding

When called, as an emergency, to a woman with vaginal bleeding, always remember to consider the possibility that the woman may be pregnant.

The important diagnosis to *exclude* is an ectopic pregnancy.

Ectopic pregnancy

- Missed or light period ± unilateral pain ± positive pregnancy test.
- Abdominal examination: ± tender in iliac fossa.
- Vaginal examination: do not undertake this unless it is likely to alter your decision to admit.

Treatment

If in any doubt about the diagnosis of an ectopic pregnancy, arrange admission. Treat shock aggressively if present (see page 10).

Threatened or inevitable miscarriage

- Missed period ± period type pains ± positive pregnancy test.
- Abdominal examination unremarkable.
- Vaginal examination: cervix open or closed.

Treatment options

1 Admission
2 Conservative.

If the bleeding is not too heavy and there is good social support consider option 2. If you do then you must remember to arrange follow up promptly. This may include ultrasonography; review by yourself or review in the hospital the following day. Also consider "Does she need anti-D immunoglobulin?" If yes, she must have it within 72 hours.

Other causes for abnormal vaginal bleeding

Pelvic inflammatory disease, complication post day procedure (for example, termination of pregnancy, D&C, colposcopy), IUCD, malignancy, cervical polyps, endometrial polyps, cervical erosion, trauma, and secondary to other causes, for example, warfarin.

Toxic shock syndrome

This syndrome can occur in menstruating women using tampons. Just remember to consider the possibility of this diagnosis. The woman may complain of a 'flu like illness, diarrhoea, vomiting, high temperature, and sometimes a sunburn like erythematous rash.

Examination will reveal a shocked patient with a diffuse erythematous rash.

Treatment

  Assess and treat **A**irway, **B**reathing, and **C**irculation
  Remove the tampon
  Arrange transfer to hospital

Ovarian hyperstimulation

This condition occurs in women who are receiving gonadotrophins for the treatment of infertility. This should be immediately obvious from the history.

Mild cases may present with a 'flu like illness, abdominal pain, nausea, and vomiting. More severe cases often have ascites and pleural effusions, and are shocked.

Treatment

  Assess and treat **A**irway, **B**reathing and **C**irculation
  Establish intravenous access and give intravenous fluids
  —start with 500 ml–1 litre of Hartmann's
  Transfer to hospital.

Obstetric emergencies

Obstetric shock

If this occurs the role of the GP is to ensure that the woman is stable and transferred to the obstetric unit.

Antepartum haemorrhage

This is bleeding after 24 weeks' gestation. If called about this problem, *treat it as a true emergency even if the woman only reports a small blood loss. There may be a large concealed blood loss. All cases* of antepartum haemorrhage require assessment by obstetricians.

The differential diagnoses are as shown in the table.

Diagnosis	Bleeding	Uterus	Ultrasonography
Abruptio placentae	Abdominal discomfort	Tender ± rock hard	
Placenta praevia	Painless	Non-tender	Low placenta
Local causes	Painless	Non-tender	Normal placenta

1 DO NOT perform a vaginal examination as this may precipitate more bleeding.
2 Despite severe shock the pulse rate may take some time to increase.
3 Establish intravenous access with the largest available cannula and treat shock aggressively if present (see page 10).
4 If available, consider calling the flying squad.

Other causes of shock in the obstetric patient

Pulmonary embolism, septicaemia, ruptured uterus *(can occur in last few weeks of pregnancy as well as in labour)*, amniotic fluid embolism *(during or just after delivery)*, and finally non-pregnancy causes.

Pre-eclampsia and eclampsia

Remember that eclampsia can occur before, during, or shortly after delivery.

Pre-eclampsia can occur any time after 20 weeks or even earlier in association with a hydatidiform mole. Most cases, however, occur after 28 weeks. The woman may notice swelling of her hands, face, ankles, or feet. Examination may reveal the classic triad of signs:

1 BP > 140/90
   or systolic BP ↑ > 30 mm Hg of booking value
   or diastolic BP ↑ > 20 mm Hg of booking value
2 Oedema of hands, face, and pre-tibia
3 Proteinuria.

It is not, however, necessary to have all these. The presence of isolated hypertension or isolated proteinuria in pregnancy should be regarded with suspicion. Oedema is non-specific and occurs in 40% of pregnancies—it is more significant if it is severe and/or still present in the morning. In the presence of mild hypertension without proteinuria, referral should be considered for assessment of the fetus.

Symptoms of *imminent eclampsia* include any of the following: headache, epigastric pain, vomiting, visual disturbances, or flashing lights.

Examination will show hyperreflexia with ankle clonus.

Treatment for pre-eclampsia and imminent eclampsia

- Arrange admission.
- Keep the woman quiet avoiding noises and bright lights.
- If the woman starts to fit:
     assess the **A**irway, **B**reathing and **C**irculation, and remember to lay her on her left side if possible
     give diazepam 10 mg i.v. (may need repeat dose).

Labour

Even though you may choose not to do home deliveries or intrapartum care you may still find yourself at a delivery. The skill required of a GP in this situation is to a level equivalent to any other GP. If you are on the obstetric list or if you undertake intrapartum care, then you will be expected to have a higher level of skill.

Normal labour (position occipital anterior)

Arrange for a midwife to meet you. If the woman is in first stage admit, if in second stage—don't panic!

Second stage
↓
Head visible
↓
Once the head is crowned, ask the woman to pant with the next contraction. To prevent uncontrolled delivery of the head, guard the occiput with the left hand and place a pad over the anus with the right hand. Apply pressure with the pad beneath the fetal chin, so allowing the perineum to sweep over the face and chin. This allows the head to be delivered slowly between contractions
↓
Slip a finger in to check the position of the cord—if around the neck slip it over the head. Aspirate baby
↓
Occiput is normally uppermost and will rotate by 90°
↓
Deliver the anterior shoulder beneath the pubic arch with the next contraction by directing the head gently down towards the bed. Give Syntometrine 1 ml i.m. (Syntocinon 5 units and ergometrine maleate 0·5 mg). Gently draw the head up to the symphysis pubis and the posterior shoulder emerges above the perineum followed by the rest of the body
↓
Suck the baby out and clamp cord after vigorous cry
↓
Keep the baby warm

Third stage
↓
If available give Syntometrine 1 ml (Syntocinon 5 units and
ergometrine maleate 0·5 mg) i.m. following delivery of the
anterior shoulder
↓
Signs of separation of the placenta:
1 the cord moves down
2 the uterus rises up
3 a small gush of blood
↓
Place one hand above symphysis pubis, applying gentle pressure
towards maternal back but also in an upward direction. Hold
umbilical cord just taut with the other
↓
Continue to hold the umbilical cord just taut. Apply gentle cord
traction downwards towards the bed at an angle of 45° from the
horizontal plane initially, rising to 45° above as the placenta
"climbs the perineum"
↓
Cord traction stops and the lower hand takes the weight of the
placenta while also rotating it so as to wind the membranes into a
rope
↓
Check placenta and membranes

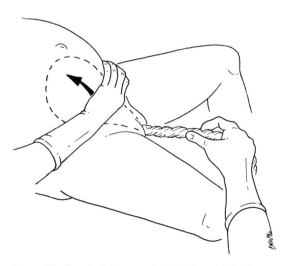

Figure 10   Brandt–Andrews method of delivery of the placenta

51

Obstetric emergencies

Notes on abnormal labour

Normal breech delivery

Exclude prolapse of the cord (see page 53)
↓
Ensure cervix is *fully* dilated
↓
Once the breech has descended to the perineum, perform an episiotomy and try to place the woman in the lithotomy position
↓
If it is a flexed breech, maternal effort should deliver the buttocks and legs
↓
If the legs are extended, flex each knee joint separately and the foot will pop out
↓
The trunk is born by descent with the flexed arms across the chest. Do not exert traction. Hold the baby by the bony pelvis, NOT the abdomen, as there is a risk to internal abdominal organs
↓
The anterior shoulder appears under the pubic arch, quickly followed by the posterior shoulder
↓
Allow the baby to hang down until the nape of the neck is visible below the pubic arch
(for a maximum of one minute)
↓
Lift the baby, by above the ankles, up to the horizontal position
↓
The head is born by the face sweeping over the perineum

Cord prolapse

Diagnosis

Suspect when there is spontaneous rupture of membranes in a breech or a transverse lie.

When a vaginal examination is performed the cord pulsations will be felt.

Management

Keep two fingers in the vagina and push the presenting part as far out of the pelvic cavity as possible. Place the woman in the knee–chest position or on all fours. Transfer to obstetric unit

General management of obstetric shock/collapse

The pregnant woman should lie on her left hand side. You can lay the woman down with pillows under her right side, or move the uterus to the left by manual displacement. This relieves pressure on the inferior vena cava and improves venous return and cardiac output.

Give the highest available concentration of oxygen. Beware the risk of regurgitation of gastric contents.

Establish intravenous access using the biggest cannula you can in the largest accessible vein. Give 500–1000 ml of Hartmann's solution to start with. Hypovolaemia is common and may result from hidden blood loss.

Postpartum emergencies

Postpartum haemorrhage

Postpartum haemorrhage (PPH) can either be primary (within 24 hours of delivery) or secondary (more than 24 hours after delivery).

Primary PPH

This is caused by bleeding from the placental site or from local lacerations. This usually requires readmission.

Secondary PPH

There are two main causes of secondary PPH—retained products and infection. The two causes may coexist. If the bleeding is severe, the woman will need to be admitted for ultrasonography and may require an evacuation of retained products of conception (ERPC) in addition to antibiotics. Before admission assess **A**irway, **B**reathing and **C**irculation.

If the bleeding is not severe, the cervical os is closed, and the uterus is involuting, then the initial management should be antibiotics including anaerobic cover. If the bleeding does not respond, then refer.

Postpartum infection

Pyrexia in a postpartum woman—defined as an isolated recording of $\geqslant 38°C$ or a reading of $37.4°C$ on three consecutive days—should be treated seriously and a cause sought.

Causes

Genital tract infection, urinary tract infection, acute mastitis, abdominal wound infection after caesarean section, chest infection after general anaesthesia, thrombophlebitis, deep vein thrombosis, pulmonary embolism, and finally any non-pregnancy-related causes, for example, viral illness, appendicectomy.

Neonatal resuscitation

Babies have a habit of appearing without warning, and some need a little help getting going. The basic principles of neonatal resuscitation are simple:

- Keep the baby warm
- Keep the baby pink
- Keep your head.

You do not need much equipment to perform basic neonatal resuscitation, and this section will remind you what to do. The most important drug is oxygen, and once again we would encourage you to carry this with you. Advanced neonatal resuscitation is difficult to perform out of hospital, although it may be worth trying and we have included the essential information here.

Apgar scores are of questionable value in general practice, but the scoring system gives an indication of how to assess a neonate, and may be relevant medicolegally.

Score	2	1	0
Colour	Pink	Blue	White
Heart rate	>100	<100	0–50 and falling
Respiration	Good cry	Weak	Absent
Tone	Active/flexed	Reduced	Flaccid
Irritability	Cry	Grimace	None

An apgar of 8–10 is OK, a score of 4–7 implies a degree of resuscitation is needed, and a score of 3 or less may mean you have a serious problem on your hands.

Basic neonatal resuscitation

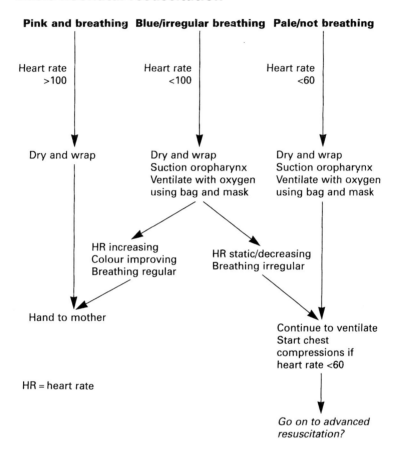

Pink and breathing

Heart rate
>100

Dry and wrap

Blue/irregular breathing

Heart rate
<100

Dry and wrap
Suction oropharynx
Ventilate with oxygen
using bag and mask

Pale/not breathing

Heart rate
<60

Dry and wrap
Suction oropharynx
Ventilate with oxygen
using bag and mask

HR increasing
Colour improving
Breathing regular

HR static/decreasing
Breathing irregular

Hand to mother

Continue to ventilate
Start chest
compressions if
heart rate <60

HR = heart rate

Go on to advanced
resuscitation?

Advanced neonatal resuscitation

Airway

The most important objective is to maintain the baby's oxygenation. Suction is essential and bag–valve–mask ventilation can be very effective. If you feel sufficiently confident, and intubation is required, do so under direct vision with a laryngoscope. In this situation it may be better to use a shouldered tube rather than an uncuffed one, to help you get the distance through the cords correct.

Breathing

Ventilate using oxygen (3–4 l/min). You must have a system with a pressure relief circuit. *Never* ventilate a baby by connecting it directly to an oxygen cylinder, because this can cause barotrauma. Ventilate at 30–40 breaths/min. Check for symmetrical chest movement and bilateral air entry.

Circulation

Perform chest compressions if the heart rate is less than 60. The rate is 120/min. Use the encircling technique (see page 8).

Epinephrine (adrenaline)

This can be given via the endotracheal tube, intravenously, or via the umbilical vein. It is accepted that none of these routes is easy to achieve in general practice.

- The endotracheal dose is 1·0 ml of 1:10 000. The counsel of perfection is to squirt it down a catheter passed through the tube.
- The intravenous dose is 0·1 ml/kg of 1:10 000 first time, or 1·0 ml/kg thereafter (every 3–5 min).

Fracture treatment

If associated with other injuries, ensure help is on its way (you or someone else has dialled 999). See page 35 for the management of major trauma. Treat according to the priorities.

Airway with immobilisation of cervical spine

- Clear the airway and open using a jaw thrust or chin lift manoeuvre
- Immobilise the neck in a neutral position (neither flexed nor hyperextended) (see page 76).

Breathing

- Ensure adequate and supplement with oxygen.

Circulation with haemorrhage control

- Establish intravenous access (preferably in a large vein such as the antecubital fossa) and give intravenous fluids (for example, Hartmann's) if needed
- Use direct pressure rather than a tourniquet to control external haemorrhage
- Be aware that there can be significant concealed blood loss from fractures, especially those of the pelvis and femur. Hypotension is rarely caused by a head injury (except in very young babies), so if present look for other injuries.

Analgesia

Intramuscular diclofenac or opiates are good for isolated limb injuries. Otherwise use intravenous opiates in small doses, repeated as required.

History of injury

Ascertain the mechanism of injury because this will give you some idea of the forces involved and the likelihood of a fracture. Be aware of transmission of forces: a fall on the outstretched hand may cause a fracture anywhere from the hand to the clavicle. Likewise a fall from a height can cause a fracture of any of the lower limb bones, any part of the spine, or the base of the skull.

Remember that children and elderly people can break bones with seemingly insignificant force, so if in any doubt arrange for an *x* ray.

There is no need to confirm all fractures with an *x* ray, if this will not alter subsequent management, for example, toe fractures—it is only unnecessary radiation. Skull *x* rays are rarely required after minor head injuries—basal skull fractures do not show and, if there is clinical concern, a CT scan may be more appropriate.

Fractures in children

Have a high suspicion of greenstick fractures.

A young child who won't weight bear after a fall may well have a "toddler's fracture" (spiral fracture of the tibia) often with minimal clinical signs. If in any doubt, ensure *x* rays are taken.

A young child who won't use his or her arm after a pulling mechanism of injury has most likely got a pulled elbow (the radial head pulls out of the annular ligament). *x* Rays are normal and so unnecessary. The arm can be manipulated easily by holding the child's hand and then pronating while flexing the elbow. Hold the thumb of the other hand over the radial head to feel for an underlying clunk. The child usually starts to use the arm again within about an hour, but it may take 24–36 hours.

**If you suspect non-accidental injury
ensure in-hospital assessment.**

59

Fracture treatment

Isolated limb fractures

- Immobilise as far as you are able, for example, with a sling for upper limb injuries, neighbour strapping for digits, temporary splints for lower limbs
- Give analgesia
- If you suspect a compound fracture, cover with a sterile dressing and give intravenous antibiotics if possible; tetanus cover is required
- If there is an absent pulse distal to a fracture with obvious deformity, then align the limb as far as possible and ensure urgent transfer to hospital.

Dislocations

These are not always clinically obvious—a displaced fracture can easily be mistaken for a dislocation. Fractures may also coexist with dislocations.

- Unless there is distal ischaemia, do not attempt to relocate dislocations before an *x* ray is taken as you may exacerbate the situation
- In most cases, you will not be able to give sufficient analgesia to overcome muscle spasm and relocate the joint. The only exceptions are for patella or recurrent shoulder dislocations.

Patellas usually dislocate laterally. Give good analgesia, if available, and then push the patella medially while extending the knee. It should just pop into place with relief of severe pain.

Soft tissue injuries

These can cause just as much morbidity as fractures. Many will respond very well to physiotherapy—the quicker the treatment starts, the better the end result is likely to be.

In all cases, treat according to the **RICE** regimen (**R**est for 24–48 hours, apply **I**ce regularly, use a **C**ompression bandage, for example, Tubigrip, and **E**levate the affected part to reduce swelling. The use of NSAIDs (when tolerated) is also of benefit. Gradual mobilisation should start within 48 hours of injury.

Minor head injuries

These are extremely common and the vast majority cause no long term disability. Advise regular analgesia (for example, paracetamol suspension), rest, and a period of observation, looking in particular for:

- repeated vomiting
- excessive drowsiness
- worsening of headache (or irritability) despite analgesia
- fitting
- unconsciousness
- blurred vision.

If any of the above, or if there are any other concerns about the patient, then refer to the local hospital for assessment.

Psychiatric emergencies

If you are called out to a psychiatric emergency, don't forget the basics before deciding upon your course of action. Also don't be reluctant to ask the Police to go with you if you are worried that you may be at risk.

- Take a history and do a physical examination
- Assess the risk of danger to the patient, to yourself, and to others
- If the problem is one of acute stress, try to discuss tensions and calm the situation
- Is medication appropriate?
- Should an immediate referral to the psychiatric service be considered, and will the patient accept the idea of assessment?

Informal admission is obviously more satisfactory than compulsory admission. If compulsory admission is needed it is important to have a good idea of the relevant sections of the Mental Health Act.

If you are reading this in an emergency, you should also be contacting the duty approved social worker as well as the psychiatric services. They are well trained in this field, and may be needed as part of the procedure.

The Mental Health Act 1983

To admit a patient under the Mental Health Act, you will require:

- Grounds for compulsory admission
- An application for compulsory admission
- Medical recommendations for compulsory admission.

Some definitions

Mental disorder is defined as mental illness, arrested or incomplete development of the mind, psychopathic disorder, and any other disorder or disability of the mind.

Mental illness is not defined in the act. Sexual deviancy, and drug or alcohol dependence are not themselves considered to be mental disorders. Mental disorder may, however, coexist or may result from drug or alcohol use.

Psychopathic disorder is a persistent disorder or disability of the mind (whether or not it includes significant impairment of intelligence), which results in abnormally aggressive or seriously irresponsible conduct on the part of the person concerned.

Mental impairment means that a person must suffer a significant impairment of intelligence and also have abnormally aggressive or seriously irresponsible conduct. *Severe* mental impairment is severe impairment of intelligence and social functioning associated with abnormally aggressive or seriously irresponsible conduct.

Section 2 of the Mental Health Act

Purpose

Admission for assessment.

Grounds

The patient should be:

- Detained in the interests of his or her own health or safety, or with a view to the protection of other persons
- Suffering from a mental disorder of a nature and degree that warrants the detention of the patient in hospital for assessment (or for assessment followed by treatment) for at least a limited period.

Application

This may be made by an approved social worker or by the "nearest relative". The applicant must have seen the patient within 14 days before the date of the application. It is often better to involve the social worker, as the relative you have on site may not be the "nearest relative" as defined in the Act, and because it can be distressing for families to get involved in the legal side of the process.

Medical recommendation

Two medical recommendations are needed:

- One from a practitioner approved under section 12 of the Act (usually a consultant psychiatrist)
- One from the GP or another approved doctor.

Both doctors must personally examine the patient, ideally together; not more than five days should elapse between the medical examinations. The doctors must state in writing why compulsory admission is required, using the correct form.

Notes

Compulsory detention can be for up to 28 days. Treatment is subject to the consent of the patient.

Section 3 of the Mental Health Act

Purpose

Admission for compulsory treatment.

Grounds

As for Section 2, except the type of mental disorder must be specified and of a nature or degree that warrants detention in hospital for treatment. This section can also be used in the case of mental impairment, severe mental impairment, or psychopathic disorder, if treatment is likely to alleviate or prevent deterioration in the condition of the patient.

Application

As for Section 2.

Medical recommendation

As for Section 2.

Notes

Lasts for up to six months in the first instance. Allows for compulsory treatment.

Section 4 of the Mental Health Act

Purpose

Emergency admission.

Grounds

As for Section 2.

Application

As for Section 2.

Medical recommendation

Only one medical recommendation is needed, preferably by a doctor with previous knowledge of the patient.

Notes

Admission should take place within 24 hours of application or examination. It is valid for 72 hours, and does not allow for compulsory treatment, except under common law. It should only be used in genuine emergencies where there would be an undesirable delay in obtaining a second medical recommendation, as required under Section 2.

Useful drug dosages

Haloperidol

A high potency neuroleptic which can be useful in mania and other excited states:

- Parenteral dose: 2–10 mg i.m., although severely disturbed patients may require up to 30 mg initial dose
- Oral dose: 5–10 mg repeated every 30 min until the patient is calm.

Droperidol

This is equipotent with haloperidol but more sedating and shorter acting:

- Dose: 5–10 mg i.m.

Thioridazine

This is equipotent with chlorpromazine, less sedative, and less prone to cause postural hypotension:

- Dose: 25–50 mg, titrated higher if necessary against effect.

Chlorpromazine

This is a useful, low potency neuroleptic with sedative properties. Use it with caution:

- Dose: 25–50 mg i.m., although many doctors will give up to 100 mg i.m.

These drugs are all contraindicated in the presence of coma induced by CNS depressants, bone marrow suppression, and phaeochromocytoma.

Intramuscular injection may be painful, and may cause hypotension and tachycardia—patients should remain supine for 30 min after such injections if at all possible.

Useful drug dosages for adverse drug reactions

In an oculogyric crisis, use parenteral procyclidine 5–10 mg.

For acute akathisia, use parenteral procyclidine ± diazepam 5 mg i.v.

Procyclidine is contraindicated in the presence of untreated urinary retention, closed angle glaucoma, and gastrointestinal obstruction.

Difficult situations

It is possible that you will encounter difficult situations when dealing with mentally ill patients.

Under common law any individual is entitled to apprehend and restrain a person who is mentally disordered and presents an imminent danger to himself or to others. This only applies until the immediate crisis is over, and does not allow the use of excessive force, or for treatment without the patient's consent.

The best general advice is to:

- remember the basics
- use this section to guide you on the Mental Health Act
- act reasonably, in good faith, with the patient's best interests in mind.

Epistaxis

Most cases are uncomplicated bleeds from Little's area, and they are usually easily dealt with. Bleeding from further back in the nose, or after trauma and surgery, can be difficult to arrest and may be life threatening.

Assessment

Airway

The nasal airway will be compromised, but be aware of the possibility of blood in the pharynx causing obstruction, especially in the unconscious patient.

Breathing and Circulation

If there is shock you should give oxygen if available, attempt to gain venous access, and give fluids (as described on page 10).

Stopping the bleeding

In a small epistaxis external pressure may suffice. This is performed with the patient in the upright seated position, head slightly forward. Tell the patient to spit up any blood that enters the pharynx. Apply firm pressure to the soft part of the nose below the bridge, between finger and thumb. Do not compress the bony part of the nose. Ideally you should do this yourself for 5 minutes, but a sensible patient can be instructed to do this under supervision. Place a bowl under the chin, to catch any blood that still comes out.

Merocel nasal packs

These are compressed, dehydrated sponges which can be placed into the nasal cavity. They expand inside the nose and can stop bleeding that has not responded to simple pressure. They are cheap, easy to insert, and don't take up much room to carry. Once inserted, the patient should be sent to hospital.

Merocel nasal packs can often be obtained via hospital ENT departments, as they are increasingly used for both epistaxis and postoperative packing.

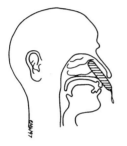

Sit the patient upright. Raise the tip of the nose while keeping the head level, and insert the Merocel 1–2 cm into the nasal cavity at an angle of about 45°

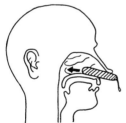

Rotate the Merocel into the horizontal plane and push it backwards into the nasal cavity, until it touches the back wall of the postnasal space. If the pack does not fully expand use 0·9% saline to rehydrate it. Tape the drawstring to the cheek

How to use a Merocel nasal pack

Nasal balloons and packing

Both of these techniques can be used in general practice, but are best suited to those with experience in their application.

Eye emergencies

The important things to check in anyone with visual problems are the following:

● presence of pupillary reaction to light
● red reflex
● visual acuity—if possible use a Snellen type chart, but at the very least assess the ability to perceive finger movement and the ability to differentiate light from dark.

Any sudden loss of vision is an emergency and should be referred immediately to the nearest hospital with ophthalmic facilities.

Artery occlusion

Sudden, painless loss of vision in one eye.

Retinal detachment

Blurred vision, often preceded by floaters and peripheral flashing lights.

Acute glaucoma

Usually presents with acutely painful, red, watering eye with greatly reduced vision. Occasionally nausea and vomiting may be the predominant symptoms, diverting attention away from the eye. The pupil is often semi-dilated, oval shaped, and with a poor light reaction. The cornea may appear cloudy and have a reduced red reflex. The eye feels hard in comparison to a normal eye.

Orbital cellulitis

Potentially sight threatening and usually requires intravenous antibiotics. Presents with very painful red discharging eye with swollen lids.

21821821821

Eye emergencies

Ophthalmic trauma

If there is disruption of the globe or an obvious penetrating injury, refer immediately. Attempts to clean or further examine the eye may exacerbate the injury. Chemical (especially alkali) burns should have expert assessment and may require prolonged irrigation. Lacerations around the eyelids, hyphaema, or a suspected intraocular foreign body all require referral.

Infections

Refer all cases of suspected acute iritis, herpes zoster, or herpes simplex infections for ophthalmic assessment.

71

Look after yourself, doctor

RTAs happen . . .

With more than 100 000 people being injured each year in speed related road accidents, each and every motorist stands a good chance of being one of the first on the scene at some time. *It could be you*, and, unlike the lottery, it probably *will* be, sooner or later. But unlike each and every motorist, you're a doctor, and you have expectations of yourself, let alone what is expected of you by others. You can't just walk away, yet even that would be better than to harm by incompetence.

To help you fulfil this unexpected and unwelcome role at the roadside, and to face parallel catastrophes in the surgery and at patients' homes, this book is designed to reduce emergency behaviour patterns to logical sequences, which can be recalled under the influence of adrenaline. We also make suggestions for what you can carry in your professional emergency equipment. If you share our dread of feeling useless and unprepared, why not ensure that you always have handy at least an airway, some surgical gloves, and a brown Venflon?

Emotional house-keeping

These days we are all aware of post-traumatic stress disorder in our patients, but don't forget the effect on yourself. Emergencies are traumatising as well as traumatic, and the doctor can feel pretty rough when life saving measures fail. We have to remember that *we can't save them all*, and to have realistic expectations of ourselves. You may need to talk it out with someone close to you, another doctor, or even an A&E consultant, to get a balanced view of the situation.

The other side of the coin is the immense satisfaction a doctor can gain by making a vital impact on the team effort to save life and minimise morbidity.

Dealing with medical emergencies is a team effort, and all the team working skills we have developed in our practice should come in useful at the scene. It's about supporting others, not criticising; about giving others space to use their skills (for example, a good paramedic knows more about cervical collars and spinal boards

72

than we do); and about being appropriately assertive when the need arises (for example, saying to the Fire Chief: *"I want him out NOW even if we damage the trapped leg, as otherwise he will die.")*. It's about taking responsibility which, after all, is what we are trained for. Nothing can train us for some of the horrors, but that's where it's about being human.

Medicolegal safety

Your professional indemnity insurance should cover you for any "Good Samaritan" acts by the roadside and in the home, whether or not you are on duty. Hippocrates and the General Medical Council demand that you attend to those who need your services; however, emergency medicine carries the same professional risks as all other aspects of practice. You must be able to refute any allegations of negligence, and the key to this is, as always, *documentation*. You keep good records of all your consultations, but did you make any notes about the RTA you attended? As part of your debrief routine after any emergency, take the time to write down some details.

DATE/TIME/NAME for example:	EVENT
	Callout and arrival on scene
	Initial assessment
	Procedures carried out
	Certification of time of death
	Transfer to hospital

At the same time as writing up your notes, you may like to think about claiming a fee from insurers under the Road Traffic Act.

RTAs are not the only emergencies ...

... But the knowledge, skills, and attitudes are transferable to many of those other terrifying situations which come out of the blue when we are least expecting them. "Doctor, doctor come quick"—a child is choking, a man has gone mad, or a woman is delivering her baby on the kitchen floor. These and countless other situations can suddenly face us. We are expected to take charge and ensure all ends well. Even if we don't actually come up against the emergency that we dread most, the potential for it to happen when we are on or off duty is enough to disturb many a GP's sleep.

It's for this reason that we have written this book. We hope that, by reading it, you will be able to think calmly and in a structured way about situations that may have been lurking in your nightmares since undergraduate days. Here is a chance to remind yourself about skills that you may never have practised and to keep up to date with the latest approaches to emergency medicine. If you spend a little time thinking about it now, it's amazing what you can recall in the heat of the moment. You don't need to be a hero, you just need to know what to do.

Hints section

How to use a coke bottle as a spacer

Spacer devices are as effective as nebulisers for drug delivery in acute asthma attacks, although the exact dosage regimen needs formal evaluation. In an emergency, and when you do not have a nebuliser, try delivering β agonists via a spacer device. In children use 8–20 puffs of salbutamol or terbutaline, delivered one puff at a time via the spacer. In adults use 10–40 puffs, one puff at a time.

An improvised spacer can be made out of a 1.5 litre plastic drinks bottle. Insert the inhaler through a hole cut in the base of the bottle, and inhale through the spout. For young children, it is possible to improvise a mask using a plastic or polystyrene drinks cup attached to the spout. An alternative in this age group is to cut the bottle in half, placing the open end over the face (watch the sharp edges). Using a coffee cup on its own as a spacer is the least effective method available.

Improvised spacers have been formally evaluated, and do work!

Finding a house in a hurry

Ask the family to leave a bucket outside by the road, to identify the correct house.

Dr Nigel Lord

It is hoped that we can expand this section with hints from readers. Any contributions will be acknowledged, and should be sent to the editors.

Practical procedures

Immobilisation of the cervical spine

Pillows, cushions, bags of intravenous fluid, rolled up newspapers, and other firm objects may all be used for immobilisation of the cervical spine. They are placed on either side of the neck beside each ear and preferably extending to just above the shoulders. Tape in place if necessary. Additional immobilisation may be provided by tape across the forehead and the chin of the patient, attaching them to the floor surface.

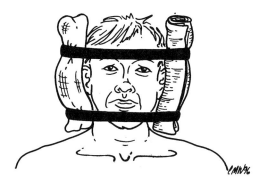

How to immobilise the cervical spine

If no equipment is available, manual immobilisation can be used to hold the neck still until the ambulance arrives with hard collars, etc.

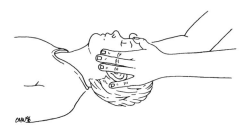

In line cervical stabilisation for manual immobilisation of the neck

How to use a defibrillator

First rule

Be familiar with the defibrillator you intend to use.

Manual defibrillator

1 Switch on
2 Select required joules
3 Remove oxygen source and GTN patches
4 Place paddles on the chest, using gel pads for contact. The positions of choice are over the right upper sternum below the clavicle and over the fifth left intercostal space—the cardiac apex
5 Press the charge button and warn that you are doing so
6 Make sure everyone is clear, then press shock buttons simultaneously
7 Recharge with the paddles on the chest or back in the unit.

Beware of water and urine.

Automatic or semi-automatic defibrillators

1 Connect the machine to the patient
2 Follow the machine's instructions.

Trouble shooting

If the machine isn't shocking and you are confident about the rhythm you wish to treat:

- If there is a manual override button or card—use it
- If the synchronised shock is on—disable it.

If you can't tell whether it's a flat line on monitor or true asystole:

- Check the leads
- Check the gain is turned up
- Check whether the machine is reading through the paddles or leads.

Notes

For children less than 10 kg use the smaller paddles. If none are available you can use adult paddles positioned at the front and back of the chest

If the patient has a pacemaker, position the paddles at least 12·5 cm away from the pacemaker.

Management of choking—practical techniques

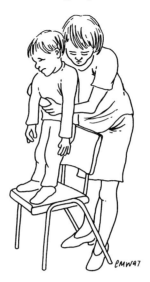

The Heimlich manoeuvre

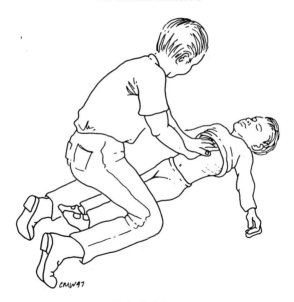

Abdominal thrusts

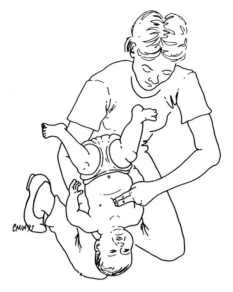

Chest thrusts in an infant

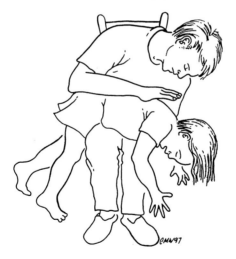

Back blows in a child

Practical procedures

Needle thoracocentesis

Used if you suspect a tension pneumothorax.

A tension pneumothorax is diagnosed if there is respiratory compromise, reduced air entry on the side of the pneumothorax, hyperresonance to percussion on the side of the pneumothorax, and a trachea deviated away from the pneumothorax. It is most common after trauma or in asthmatic individuals.

Equipment
Something to clean the skin
16 gauge or larger intravenous cannula
20 ml syringe, if possible with a three way tap

Procedure

1 Identify the second intercostal space in the midclavicular line
2 Clean the chest wall
3 Attach the syringe to the cannula
4 Insert the cannula at 90° to the chest wall, just above the third rib, aspirating as you go
5 If air is aspirated remove the syringe and needle, leaving the plastic cannula in place with the hub end open to the atmosphere
6 Secure the cannula where it enters the chest. It will need to stay there until a chest drain is inserted in hospital

There is a 10–20% chance of causing a simple pneumothorax in a patient on whom this procedure is attempted, and who does not have a tension pneumothorax. That is OK; there is a greater chance of dying from a tension pneumothorax.

The second intercostal space lies below the second rib. The second rib is the first rib you can feel beneath the clavicle, and articulates with the sternum at the sternal angle (the ridge in the sternum). Go above the third rib, rather than below the second rib, to avoid the neurovascular bundle.

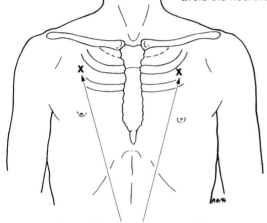

Second intercostal space, mid-clavicular line

Needle thoracocentesis—finding the second intercostal space

Needle cricothyroidotomy

Used if you suspect airway obstruction above the level of the cricothyroid membrane. Have you tried simple airway clearing/opening manoeuvres first? Can you intubate?

This is not an easy procedure in children—be especially careful of the anatomy.

Equipment
Something to clean the skin
Large intravenous cannula (16 gauge or larger)
5 or 10 ml syringe
Three way tap or Y connector if possible
A supply of oxygen with oxygen tubing
Procedure
1 Attach the syringe to the cannula
2 Identify the cricothyroid membrane. This is best done by sliding your finger from the chin downwards until you come to a prominent bump with a dimple in the top—the thyroid cartilage. The soft bit between this cartilage, and the firm cricoid cartilage inferiorly, is the cricothyroid membrane
3 Clean the skin over the area
4 Stabilise the cricothyroid area with your left hand. Extend the neck if there is no risk of cervical spine injury
5 Insert the needle through the skin over the cricothyroid membrane. Aim the needle towards the feet at an angle of 45° to the skin, aspirating as you go
6 When air is aspirated, gently slide the cannula into trachea—take care not to damage the posterior tracheal wall
7 Remove the needle and recheck that air can be aspirated
8 If the patient can self ventilate then direct an oxygen jet over the cannula hub. If you need to ventilate the patient, connect the oxygen tubing to the cannula using the three way tap or Y connector as shown in the figure. If you don't have a connector you need to cut a small hole in the side of the tubing to act as a valve, and can try connecting the oxygen to the cannula via the barrel of a 2 ml syringe (push the tubing into the back of the barrel, and connect the cannula at the front)
9 In adults set the oxygen flow rate to 6 l/min. In children set the oxygen flow to 1 l/min per year of age. Increase flow as necessary
10 Ventilate by occluding the three way tap/Y connector/hole for one second, then releasing for four seconds to allow passive exhalation
11 Check the neck is not swelling from subcutaneous injection of gas
12 Watch for chest movement, secure the cannula, and await help

Note: passive exhalation normally occurs through the upper airway during this procedure. There is usually enough of a gap to allow the air to escape. If passive exhalation does not occur, because the upper airway is totally obstructed, it may be necessary to reduce the oxygen flow rate to 1–2 l/min. In adults another option is to insert a second cannula through the cricothyroid membrane—leaving the hub end open to the atmosphere. These measures will allow passive exhalation.
You cannot ventilate a patient through a needle cricothyroidotomy using a bag–valve–mask.

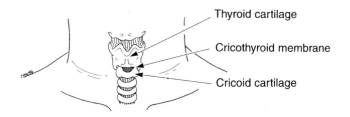

Thyroid cartilage

Cricothyroid membrane

Cricoid cartilage

How to find the cricothyroid membrane

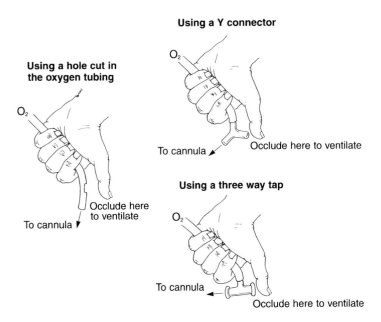

Using a Y connector

O₂

Using a hole cut in the oxygen tubing

O₂

Occlude here to ventilate

To cannula

To cannula

Occlude here to ventilate

Using a three way tap

O₂

To cannula

Occlude here to ventilate

How to ventilate the patient after a cricothyroidotomy

Using an intraosseous needle

This procedure isn't difficult, can easily be performed in the community, and can save lives. It is used in children aged less than six years. There is evidence that it can be safely and effectively utilised after only a short period of training. Such training can be obtained from the specialised courses detailed elsewhere, or perhaps from your local A&E department.

Equipment
Something to clean the skin
Intraosseous needle (much preferred) or 16 gauge cannula at least 1·5 cm in length
20 ml syringe filled with 0·9% saline, ideally with a short extension set and three way tap
Infusion fluid

Procedure
1 Identify the infusion site. Avoid fractured bones, or limbs with proximal fractures. If possible avoid areas of infected burns or cellulitis
   Proximal tibia: anteromedial surface, 2–3 cm below the tibial tuberosity
   Distal tibia proximal to the medial malleolus
   Distal femur: midline, 2–3 cm above the epicondyles
2 Prepare the skin
3 Insert the needle through the skin, and perpendicularly/slightly away from the growth plate into the bone with a screwing motion. There is a give as the marrow cavity is entered
4 Unscrew the trocar and confirm position by aspirating bone marrow or by flushing with 5–10 ml 0·9% saline (marrow cannot always be aspirated, but it should flush easily)
5 Secure the needle and splint the limb
Fluids can be infused through an intraosseous needle as through a standard intravenous cannula. If rapid fluid replacement is required, infuse under pressure using a 50 ml syringe. Dilute strong alkalis and hypertonic solutions. **After giving a drug through an intraosseous needle—flush it through.**
Contraindications: proximal ipsilateral fracture; ipsilateral vascular injury; osteogenesis imperfecta; osteoporosis.
Complications: failure to enter the bone marrow—extravasation or subperiosteal infusion; osteomyelitis is rare in short term use. Local infection, skin necrosis, pain, compartment syndrome, fat and bone marrow microemboli all reported, but these are rare and if you are doing this in general practice the child really needs it!

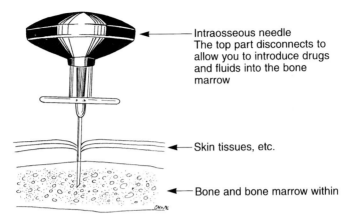

Intraosseous needle
The top part disconnects to
allow you to introduce drugs
and fluids into the bone
marrow

Skin tissues, etc.

Bone and bone marrow within

Using an intraosseous needle

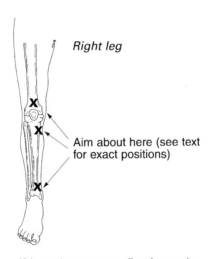

Right leg

Aim about here (see text
for exact positions)

Using an intraosseous needle: where to aim

Pulse oximetry

Pulse oximeters are becoming an increasingly common sight in pre-hospital care. Some GPs use them, and some ambulances may carry them. It is as well to know a little about them.

A pulse oximeter is a combined red and infrared light source with a detector. You clip the probe on a finger or toe and get a reading of the patient's pulse rate and oxyhaemoglobin saturation. If the machine has a tone it will vary with pulse and saturation.

These machines are useful because cyanosis is not clinically detectable above an oxygen saturation of 80%, but the patient may be hypoxaemic. The alarms on pulse oximeters are usually set at 90%, and oxygen should usually be administered when the saturation falls below this.

Sources of error include poor circulation, movement, external light, nail varnish, and dyes. These machines are unreliable in carbon monoxide poisoning.

A compact device no larger than a box of matches is now available. It costs around £400.

Endotracheal administration of drugs

This is the least effective method of drug delivery but is better than nothing. It is only used if you cannot get intravenous access at a cardiac arrest, but the patient has been succesfully intubated

- Epinephrine (adrenaline) and atropine can be administered via an endotracheal tube. Give either (1) via a catheter positioned through and beyond the end of the tube or (2) by instilling the drug, diluted to 1–10 ml in 0·9% saline, directly into the tube—followed by a flush of 1–5 ml 0·9% saline, thereafter hyperventilating the patient.
- It is generally recommended to double drug dosages when giving drugs via this route.

Further information and training

Resuscitation and emergency medical care are practically based skills which are infrequently used in general practice, but where it is important to perform well and keep up to date.

All GPs should endeavour to refresh their cardiopulmonary resuscitation (CPR) and defibrillation skills on a yearly basis. This can be variously arranged through the local ambulance service, hospital, or postgraduate education programme.

We would recommend GPs who regularly take part in roadside trauma care, or who have an interest in pre-hospital emergency care, to obtain further training on an appropriate course. The British Association for Immediate Care (BASICS) is a voluntary organisation which aims to foster and improve the provision of immediate care in the community. Its members provide medical help in conjunction with emergency services at the scene of an accident or emergency. BASICS runs a Pre-Hospital Emergency Care course, and an Immediate Care course.

Joan Clark, Chief Executive
BASICS
7 Black Horse Lane
Ipswich, Suffolk IPI 2EF
Tel. 01473 218407

- The Faculty of Pre-Hospital Care also provides advanced training, for instance through its Diploma in Immediate Medical Care (tel. 0131 527 1600).
- Pre-hospital and Advanced Trauma Life Support courses are also held in the UK through the Royal College of Surgeons (tel. 0171 405 3474).
- Pre-hospital Paediatric Life Support courses are held by the Advanced Life Support Group (tel. 0161 877 1999).
- The Advanced Life Support in Obstetrics training courses are held as part of the Maternal and Neonatal Training project, and are GP friendly (tel. 01665 575386).

What to carry in your doctor's bag

We have included a comprehensive list of what you might consider carrying, and have tried to present the lists in such a way as to simplify the "what is relevant to me?" thought processes. These are suggestions only.

You will need an appropriate case, where everything is easily accessible. It is important to check regularly that your drug stock is in date. A practice or deputising service resuscitation kit, passed from doctor to doctor, can minimise outlay on expensive and/or rarely used drugs and equipment.

If you choose to carry more advanced equipment, ensure that it is compatible with that carried by the local ambulance service. It is worth talking to them before buying anything—ask if they have any spares and you may be offered them! Do not forget to update your skills.

If you need further advice on tried and tested equipment you can contact the BASICS equipment committee (address on page 87).

Basic equipment

- Stethoscope
- Sphygmomanometer
- Auroscope/ophthalmoscope and spare batteries
- Thermometer set (normal, rectal, low reading)
- Tongue depressors
- Pinnard stethoscope/Doppler
- Tendon hammer
- Pregnancy wheel
- Peak flow meter, mouthpieces, predicted peak flow chart
- Pentorch
- Tape measure

- BM strips and stylets, or Glucometer
- Urinalysis strips
- Urine/specimen pots, swabs, bacteriology forms
- Blood bottles and forms
- Syringes and needles
- Tourniquet
- Sharps bin
- Disposable gloves and lubricating jelly
- Scissors

- Note paper and envelopes
- Prescription pads (NHS and private)
- *x* Ray forms
- Physiotherapy request forms
- GMS forms
- Maps
- BNF
- Strong torch
- *What to do in a General Practice Emergency*

What to carry in your doctor's bag

Basic kit

Useful if you don't want to carry too much, but want to have most problems covered. Assumes the local ambulance service has a fast response time, and well trained and equipped crew

Airway, Breathing and Circulation management

nebuliser (or at the very least a spacer device)
pocket mask
oropharyngeal airways of various sizes
Venflons of various sizes
Alcowipes/iodine wipes

Drugs

epinephrine 1 mg/ml, 1:1000 (need enough to give a 5 mg dose)
atropine 1 mg/10 ml (need enough to give a 3 mg dose)
50% glucose, 50 ml
glucagon 1 mg injection
Hypostop gel
chlorpheniramine 10 mg/1 ml
hydrocortisone 100 mg for injection (need enough to give
    200 mg)
diazepam 10 mg rectal tubes
diazepam emulsion 10 mg/2 ml
frusemide 50 mg/5 ml or bumetanide 5 mg/10 ml
Syntometrine injection 1 ml ampoule
aspirin 300 mg tablets
paracetamol 125 mg suppositories
co-proxamol tablets
ibuprofen 200 mg tablets or equivalent
diclofenac 75 mg injection
pethidine 100 mg/2 ml
diamorphine 10 mg injection (or morphine sulphate)
metoclopramide 10 mg/2 ml
metoclopramide 10 mg tablets
amoxycillin 250 mg/500 mg capsules
amoxycillin 500 mg dispersible tabs or 125 mg Fiztabs

erythromycin 250 mg tablets
flucloxacillin 250 mg capsules
trimethoprim 200 mg tablets
metronidazole 400 mg tablets
benzylpenicillin 600 mg injection (carry enough to give 1200 mg)
chloramphenicol eye ointment 1% or neomycin eye ointment
    0·5%
salbutamol 2·5 mg nebules
atrovent 250 μg nebules
salbutamol 100 μg inhaler
prednisolone 5 mg soluble tablets
GTN spray
frusemide 20 mg tablets
prochlorperazine 5 mg tablets
cetirizine 10 mg tablets
temazepam 10 mg tablets
chlorpromazine 10 mg tablets
chlorpromazine 50 mg/2 ml or equivalent
glycerol suppositories, adult
water for injections 2 ml and 10 ml ampoules
0·9% saline for injections 10 ml ampoules
local anaesthetic (prilocaine is increasingly used in preference to
    lignocaine)

Other bits and pieces

gauze pads
bandages
tape
Elastoplast roll
sling
safety pins
dressing pack
Steri-Strips
sodium chloride or chlorhexidine solution
sterile gloves
bags to clear up

What to carry in your doctor's bag

Intermediate kit and beyond

This is designed to offer more comprehensive treatment options and alternatives. Dip into it as you want. This would be the sort of kit you may need if you are further away from ambulance services/hospitals, or have special interest in pre-hospital care. *Contains everything in the basic kit plus the following:*

Airway, Breathing and Circulation management

oxygen with delivery set and mask
suction device ± mucus extractor
2 × blood giving sets
Hartmann's solution
three way tap

Drugs

paracetamol 500 mg soluble tablets
codydramol tablets
nefopam 30 mg tablets
codeine phosphate 30 mg tablets
diclofenac 50 mg suppositories
pethidine 50 mg tablets
MST (morphine) 10 mg tablets
amethocaine 0·5% eye drops (single use units)
migraine relief preparation (for example, sumatriptan)
erythromycin 125 mg granules
co-amoxiclav 375 mg tablets
cefaclor 375 mg modified release tablets
doxycycline 100 mg capsules
ciprofloxacin 250 mg tablets
clotrimazole pessary 500 mg
ipratropium bromide 20 µg inhaler
prochlorperazine 5 mg suppositories or domperidone 30 mg
    suppositories
loperamide capsules 2 mg
hyoscine butylbromide 10 mg tablets
antacid tablets

92

oral rehydration salt sachets
glycerol suppositories, child
diazepam 2 mg tablets
emergency contraception (for example, PC4 pack)
nizatidine 300 mg capsules
isosorbide mononitrate 20 mg tablets
digoxin 125 μg tablets
enemas (for example, Micralax)
lignocaine gel

Other bits and pieces

non-adherent dressing
big pads
clear dressing
cotton wool roll
instruments (needle holders, scalpel, mosquito/toothed forceps)
sutures
nasal pack
small torniquet for digits
umbilical cord clamps
obstetric pack

And for completeness

defibrillator
laryngoscope, endotracheal tubes, and Magill's forceps
nasopharyngeal airways
intraosseous needle and short extension set
aminophylline 250 mg/10 ml
cefotaxime 1 g injection or ceftriaxone 1 g injection
procyclidine 10 mg/2 ml

Modular kits

These are not prioritised. Dip into them as you wish.

Resuscitation kit

Airway, Breathing and Circulation management
nebuliser
oxygen with delivery set and mask
suction device ± mucus extractor
pocket mask
oropharyngeal airways of various sizes
laryngoscope, endotracheal tubes, and Magill's forceps
Venflons (selection from pink to brown)
intraosseous needle with short extension set and three way tap
2 × blood giving sets
Hartmann's solution
syringes
needles
Alcowipes/iodine wipes
tape

Drugs
epinephrine 1 mg/ml, 1:1000 (need enough to give a 5 mg dose)
atropine 1 mg/10 ml (need enough to give a 3 mg dose)
50% glucose, 50 ml
glucagon 1 mg injection
chlorpheniramine 10 mg/1 ml
hydrocortisone 100 mg for injection (need enough to give 200 mg)
diazepam 10 mg rectal tubes
diazepam emulsion 10 mg/2 ml
frusemide 50 mg/5 ml or bumetanide 5 mg/10 ml
aminophylline 250 mg/10 ml
Syntometrine injection 1 ml ampoule
naloxone 400 µg/ml
10% calcium chloride 10 ml ampoule
diamorphine or equivalent
metoclopramide 10 mg/2 ml
benzylpenicillin 600 mg injection (enough to give 1200 mg)
GTN spray
water for injection 2 ml and 10 ml ampoules
salbutamol 2.5 mg and atrovent 250 µg for the nebuliser
0·9% saline for injection 10 ml ampoules

Other bits and pieces
defibrillator
dressing pack
gauze
gloves
sharps bin
bags to clear up

Kit for dealing with trauma
strong torch
gloves
warning triangle
fluorescent waistcoat
space blanket
stethoscope
oxygen with giving set and mask
suction device
airways (oropharyngeal/nasopharyngeal)
Venflons
intraosseous needles with short extension set and three way tap
two blood giving sets
Hartmann's solution—carry 2 litres
Micropore
dressing pack
skin marker
diamorphine or equivalent with antiemetic
local anaesthetic (prilocaine is increasingly being used in
    preference to lignocaine)
needles, syringes
swabs
Tuf-Kut scissors or equivalent

Neonatal resuscitation kit
oxygen supply, with flowmeter and tubing
bag and mask with blow off valve and oxygen reservoir
suction device
straight bladed laryngoscope (with spare bulb and batteries)
endotracheal tubes (size 2.0 mm, 2.5 mm, 3.0 mm, 3.5 mm)
syringes and needles
fine catheter (to pass down ETT for drug administration)
epinephrine 1:10 000
a supply of warm towels from the household concerned!

Index

Index

needle cricothyroidotomy 82–3
needle thoracocentesis 80–1
neonatal resuscitation 55–7, 95
nitrous oxide 39

obstetrics
  advanced life support
    courses 87
  emergencies 48–54
  shock 48, 53
oculogyric crisis 67
ophthalmic trauma 71
opiates
  fractures 58
  myocardial infarction 16
  overdose 21
  pulmonary oedema 18
orbital cellulitis 70
oropharyngeal airway 37
ovarian hyperstimulation 47
oxygen 9, 14, 15, 27

pacemakers 77
paediatric emergencies *see* children
paracetamol 32
patella, dislocation 60
personal safety 72–4
  drowning 44
  electrocution 42
  psychiatric emergencies 62
  road traffic accidents 35
placenta, delivery 51
placenta praevia 48
pneumothorax, tension 37, 80–81
pocket mask 4, 8
poisoning 21
post-traumatic stress disorder 72
prednisolone 14, 15, 25, 27
pre-eclampsia 49
Pre-Hospital and Advanced
    Trauma Life Support
    courses 87
Pre-Hospital Paediatric Life
    Support courses 87
procyclidine 67
psychiatric emergencies 62–7
pulmonary embolism 18
pulmonary oedema 18, 40
pulse oximetry 86
pupils
  hypothermia 45

  reaction to light 70
  resuscitation 9
  unconscious patient 21

recovery position 3
red reflex 70
resuscitation 1–9
  drowning 9, 44
  hypothermia 45
  kit 94
  neonatal 55–7, 95
  refresher training 87
Resuscitation Council (UK) 1, 5
retinal artery occlusion 70
retinal detachment 70
RICE regimen 61
road traffic accidents 35–9, 72

salbutamol
  anaphylaxis 13, 25
  asthma 14, 15, 27
  spacer devices 75
seizures 19
  children 32
shock 10–11
  anaphylactic 13, 25
  children 10, 11, 23, 25, 28
  obstetric 48, 53
  septic 28
soft tissue injuries 61
spacer devices, improvised 75
steroids 13, 14, 15, 25
stridor 29
Syntometrine 50, 51

terbutaline 14, 15, 27, 75
tetanus 41
thioridazine 66
thoracocentesis, needle 80–1
thrombolysis 17
toxic shock syndrome 47
trauma kit 95
triage 36

uterus, ruptured 48

vaginal bleeding 46–7
ventilation
  after cricothyroidotomy 83
  neonates 57

x rays 59